WARRIORS OF THE MIND

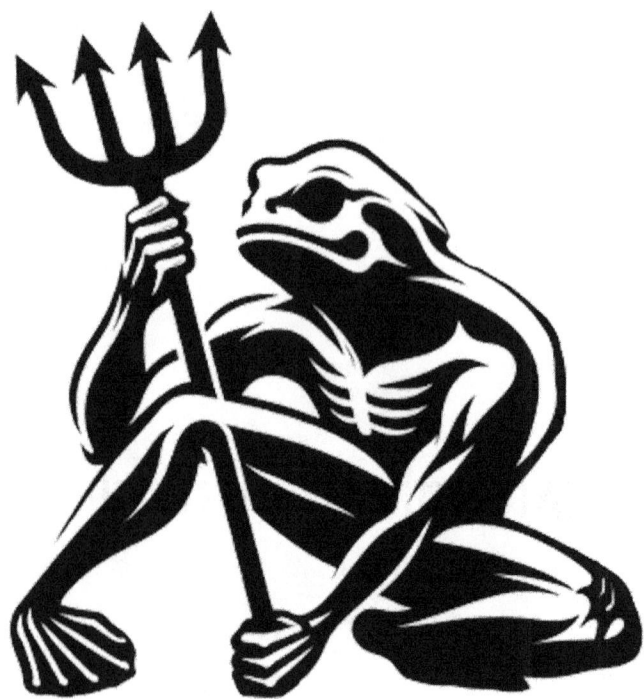

WARRIORS OF THE MIND

A Guide to Psychedelic-Assisted Psychotherapy for Combat Veterans & Their Families

DR. DAVE FERRUOLO

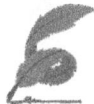

Dr. Dave Books

Dr. Dave Books
PO BOX 6421
Laconia, NH 03247
drdavebooks.com

Warriors of the Mind: A Guide to Psychedelic-Assisted Psychotherapy for
Combat Veterans & Their Families

ISBN: 978-0-9776412-4-6 (paperback)

Printed in the USA
0 1 2 3 4 5 6 7 8 9

First Printing, 2024

DISCLAIMER

PLEASE READ

For Informational Purposes Only This book, "Warriors of the Mind: A Guide to Psychedelic- Assisted Psychotherapy for Combat Veterans & Their Families," is intended solely as an informational guidebook. The journey you're about to embark upon is akin to preparing for a challenging hike through unfamiliar terrain. Just as one would need a map and guidance from seasoned experts, this book seeks to navigate you through the complex landscape of psychedelic- assisted psychotherapy. It is not a manual for self-treatment, nor should it be used as a standalone tool for diagnosing or treating psychological conditions.

Legal Implications Venturing into the realm of psychedelics can be as fraught with legal considerations as navigating through a minefield. It is crucial to be aware of and adhere to the legal framework governing the use of such substances. This book does not endorse or encourage any activities that fall outside the parameters of the law. The administration of psychedelic substances for therapeutic purposes must be conducted under the supervision of healthcare professionals within the legal boundaries of your jurisdiction. The author and publisher disclaim any responsibility for the unlawful use or possession of any substances discussed.

Safety Implications Like the unpredictability of a high-altitude climb, psychedelic substances have powerful and variable effects on both mind and body. Potential risks include adverse psychological reactions, potent interactions with other medications, and a possibility of misuse. It is imperative that any therapeutic use of psychedelics be supervised by medical professionals in a controlled environment. This book's discussions on the therapeutic potential of psychedelics are not endorsements for self-administration.

Importance of Professional Help As a meticulously built shelter provides safety in a storm, professional medical and psychological treatment offers protection and guidance through the tempest of mental health challenges. If you or a family member are facing issues such as PTSD, moral injury, or substance use disorders, it is essential to seek individualized treatment from qualified professionals. This book is a starting point for understanding, not a substitute for professional healthcare.

Individual Results May Vary Just as every musician's interpretation of a score is unique, so too are individual responses to therapy, including psychedelic-assisted psychotherapy. The information within these pages draws from a body of research, clinical trials, and therapeutic experiences, which may not necessarily predict or guarantee any specific personal outcome.

Limitation of Liability Navigating the complexities of mental health is akin to repairing a sophisticated engine; it requires expert knowledge and precision. The author and publisher are not the mechanics in this scenario, but rather the providers of a manual. They shall not be liable for any damage that may arise from the interpretation or use of the information provided. You, the reader, are encouraged to approach this book as you would a compass—a tool for guidance, not an infallible GPS

ACCEPTANCE OF TERMS

FORWARD

THE QUEST FOR HEALING PSYCHEDELICS AND THE COMBAT VETERAN'S JOURNEY

The war-torn psyche, with its depth of scars, often bears the burden of experiences that language fails to encapsulate. Combat veterans returning from the theater of war frequently find themselves trapped in the snares of PTSD, moral injury, and substance use—a trinity of afflictions that conventional therapies often address with limited success. In this milieu of healing and hope, psychedelics emerge not as a cure-all but as a profound key to a realm of therapeutic possibilities hitherto uncharted by many.

Why psychedelics, one might ask? The answer lies not in the escapism that these substances are unfairly caricatured as facilitating but in their unique ability to facilitate a therapeutic reconquest of the self. These substances, when used under the meticulous guidance of trained professionals,

offer a passage through the mind's defenses, allowing veterans to confront and integrate traumatic memories in a manner that traditional therapies often fail to achieve.

The success of psychedelics in psychotherapy is not an anecdotal tale; empirical evidence supports the efficacy. Studies have shown that substances like psilocybin and MDMA can catalyze profound emotional and cognitive transformations, particularly in individuals with recalcitrant PTSD. By disrupting the default mode network, the neurological seat of the ego, psychedelics provide veterans a rare opportunity for a psychological sortie, an insurgence against the entrenched patterns of negative thought and reliving of past horrors.

From a multidisciplinary perspective, the use of psychedelics as therapeutic agents is a convergence of medicine, psychology, spirituality, and philosophy. This synergy speaks to the warrior's soul, integrating Eastern contemplative practices that have long recognized the value of altered states of consciousness with Western psychotherapeutic modalities. The result is a holistic approach that acknowledges the multifaceted nature of the healing process.

For combat veterans, the therapeutic journey with psychedelics is an experience that promises a return to a semblance of wholeness. It is a testament to their courage that they embark on this journey, not on the battlegrounds they are accustomed to but within the uncharted territories of the mind. Here, in the depths of consciousness, they encounter the shadows of war and the potential for peace and reintegration into the civilian life that awaits their return.

Within this context, the therapist acts not as a mere observer but as a guide, a fellow traveler well-versed in the terrain of the psyche. The presence of such a guide is crucial, for they serve as the compass that helps navigate the turbulent waters of the subconscious, ensuring that the therapeutic potential of psychedelics is fully realized and integrated into the veteran's ongoing narrative.

The discussion surrounding psychedelics for combat veterans is not a mere academic exercise but an urgent call to expand our therapeutic horizons. As we stand on the precipice of a new era in psychotherapy, we must approach this frontier with an open mind and a steadfast commitment to the well-being of those who have borne the battle. For the veteran who has traversed the desolation of war, psychedelics offer not an escape but a gateway to healing—a chance to author a new chapter in their lives, one where peace and mental fortitude are once again within reach.

CONTENTS

Introduction

Welcome to *Warriors of the Mind: A Guide to Psychedelic-Assisted Psychotherapy for Combat Veterans & Their Families.* If you're reading this book, you likely belong to a unique fraternity forged through the trials of war—a fraternity that understands the meaning of service, courage, and sacrifice. Yet, even as warriors of body and mind, many of you may find yourselves embroiled in battles of a different sort: emotional and psychological skirmishes that are less visible but no less grueling than physical combat.

The purpose of this book is multifaceted. First and foremost, it serves as a navigational tool for combat veterans who are grappling with emotional and psychological issues in their post-combat lives— be it PTSD, moral injury, or substance use disorders. Here, you will find scientifically-grounded and empathetic guidance tailored to your unique experiences and challenges.

Additionally, this book is a resource for close family members who love and support veterans. As someone who has been at the forefront of caregiving, you'll find that the impact of war doesn't only reverberate through the individuals who've been deployed; it sends shockwaves through the entire family unit. Understanding the potential therapeutic value of psychedelics can be as transformative for family members as it is for veterans themselves, aiding in mutual growth and the deepening of familial bonds.

Leveraging a blend of perspectives, from medicine and psychology to spirituality and philosophy—both Eastern and Western—this guide aims to be a comprehensive manual on psychedelic-assisted psychotherapy. We don't stop at merely presenting the facts; we delve into the complex arrays of the human psyche rooted in the unique experience of combat veterans and their families.

The author of *Warriors of the Mind* combines his military background as a former Navy SEAL with professional credentials in psychology and psychotherapy. This unique vantage point enables a nuanced, deeply empathetic, and rigorously scientific understanding. His research and experience with the healing power of psychedelics add a practical layer to the theoretical scaffolding, offering real-world applications to the insights you will gain.

This book aims to challenge your beliefs, provoke deep introspection, and inspire transformative change. While we venture into profound and often heavy topics, *Warriors of the Mind* will often incorporate wit and levity to balance the emotional weight. You will also find poignant anecdotes illuminating key points, making the scientific and philosophical discussions relatable and engaging.

However, it's crucial to underscore that this book is not a substitute for professional medical or psychological care. Readers are strongly encouraged to consult healthcare professionals for diagnoses and treatments tailored to individual needs.

Whether you are a combat veteran, a loving family member, or someone invested in the well-being of these warriors of the mind, this book is for you. Let's journey to a newfound understanding, healing, and a rich, fulfilling life.

Welcome, warriors of the mind. Your quest for inner peace and healing begins here.

PART I

The Reality of Combat and the Aftermath

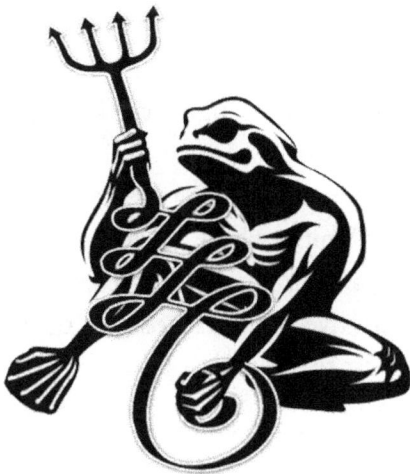

CHAPTER 1

The Combat Experience: A Primer

The theater of war paints a starkly different landscape than any encountered in the realms of civilian life. Its terrain is one of the soul as much as of the earth—a place where the skies are laden with more than the weight of weather, and the ground resonates with more than the tremors of nature. Here, the true mettle of warriors is forged and fractured.

In the framework of combat, the immediate moment dominates everything: a present thick with the dust of explosions, the smell of spent gunpowder, and the cacophony of orders cutting through the clamor. To survive, the warrior becomes hyper-attuned to this turbulent environment, their senses sharpened to a razor's edge. Yet, amidst the chaos, a silent thread weaves through—the knowledge that each action and decision bears weight beyond measure.

In this vast and often unforgiving theater, consider the journey of Navy SEAL operator Smith, whose service took him from the treacherous streets of Mogadishu to the sun-scorched earths of Iraq and Afghanistan. His narrative is one etched into the fabric of his being, a tale of resilience amidst the relentless unpredictability of guerrilla warfare and urban combat.

Mogadishu was a different kind of horror—a city where urban warfare brought combat into claustrophobic proximity. Smith's SEAL platoon navigated through narrow alleys and dense markets, where the distinction between civilian and combatant was blurred by necessity and survival. In these close quarters, the immediacy of danger was constant, and the stakes of leadership weighed heavily upon him. The sense of responsibility for his team's lives fused with the overarching mission, driving home the relentless pressure that shapes the psyche of a commander.

The Middle East presented a landscape of contrasts: rugged beauty juxtaposed against the daily reality of deadly threats. Smith's platoon confronted arduous mountain terrain, where every rock and shadow could conceal an enemy. The rules of engagement were as complex as the terrain, demanding a balance between tactical precision and ethical clarity. Smith often found himself reflecting on the delicate interplay between the warrior's code and the human spirit, contemplating the toll each decision takes on the soul of a soldier.

Smith's experiences embody the complexity of modern warfare, where soldiers must be as adept in philosophical fortitude as they are in physical combat. His service in these diverse environments speaks to the adaptability and resilience required of our SEALs. It offers a glimpse into the profound challenges faced by those who operate in the shadowed corners of conflict.

In reflecting upon the experiences of modern combat veterans, we must not lose sight of those who came before—the veterans of Vietnam, Grenada, Panama, and other conflicts that may not dominate today's headlines but still echo in the lives of those who served. These individuals have shouldered their burdens through decades, long before our society began to grapple with the complexities of their return to civilian life. Their battles did not conclude upon their departure from foreign soil; instead, they have carried the war within them, often in silence, without the framework or support systems we are striving to build now.

The wars of the past may differ in the landscapes, politics, and technologies that defined them, but the warriors share a common thread—a thread spun from duty, sacrifice, and the toll that combat extracts from the human spirit. Vietnam veterans returned to a world that was frequently indifferent or even hostile to their service. They have lived with their memories and scars, both visible and invisible, with a resilience that commands our most profound respect.

This section of our guide does not shy away from the rugged truths of the combat experience. It seeks to provide clarity and understanding to veterans and their families, elucidating the psychological and emotional topography of warfare. By doing so, we aim to facilitate a bridge back to a world where hypervigilance is no longer the norm, where the sound of fireworks doesn't evoke the reflexes honed in battle, and where the warrior can find a semblance of peace in a society that has not shared their experiences but is willing to extend a hand of support.

As we delve into the shadows cast by war, our goal is to throw light upon paths that lead out of darkness, offering insights and therapeutic avenues—such as the thoughtful application of psychedelics in a clinical setting—to guide the journey home in body, mind and spirit. With this foundational understanding of the combat experience, we can appreciate the profound transformations required in the aftermath and offer tools for healing and hope.

The Physiology of Combat

The interplay between the body and mind in the theater of combat is a symphony of survival instincts orchestrated by millennia of evolutionary biology. When a soldier steps into the cauldron of war, the body's physiology adapts in real-time, responding to the visceral reality of threat with profound changes that ripple through every system.

This adrenalized state of existence goes beyond heightened awareness. It's a holistic alteration of the body's priorities. Blood is shunted away from the digestive system to muscles primed for action. Vision may narrow, focusing intently on immediate threats while filtering out extraneous information—a phenomenon known as "tunnel vision." Hearing becomes attuned to the sounds of danger: the metallic click of a weapon's safety, the rustle of movement, or the whisper of displaced air that precedes an incoming threat.

However, while advantageous on the battlefield, these physiological changes can become persistent adversaries when the combatant returns to a non-threatening environment. The body's stress-response system, engaged intensively and repetitively, can become dysregulated. Veterans may find themselves in a chronic state of arousal, where the psychological triggers of daily life illicit the same intense physiological responses that were once necessary for survival.

This aspect of combat physiology is critical for veterans and their families to understand. It explains why seemingly innocuous stimuli—a backfiring car, a loud noise, or an unexpected touch—can trigger disproportionate reactions to the event. Recognizing these responses as relics of a once-necessary survival mechanism can be the first step to re-calibration and recovery.

In the context of psychedelic-assisted psychotherapy, understanding the physiology of combat stress is paramount. Psychedelics, when used under the guidance of a trained professional, have shown promise in re-setting the brain's response to stressors, potentially offering relief from the constant replay of the fight or flight response. This promising area of therapy, grounded in both compassion and scientific inquiry, seeks to alleviate the heavy toll that combat takes on the body long after the immediate danger has passed.

For the warriors who have returned from battle with their bodies still reverberating to the drumbeat of war, this book aims to be a bridge to a peace that encompasses both mind and body. It's a call to those who have experienced and survived combat to heal through understanding it and transforming the biological echoes of war into harmonies of health and wholeness.

Emotional and Cognitive Functioning

The emotional and cognitive functioning in combat is a delicate balancing act, a tightrope between the necessity of control and the innate human desire for emotional connection. Soldiers are trained to modulate their emotions to dial down fear and empathy when hesitation or deep feeling could mean the difference between life and death. This skill, though invaluable in the heat of combat, does not constantly recalibrate to the rhythms of civilian life.

Emotional numbing can serve as a protective barrier in a war zone, creating a shield against the full impact of traumatic events. However, this protective mechanism can persist, hindering a veteran's ability to experience a full range of emotions. Joy, sorrow, love—these fundamental human experiences can seem distant or muted, and relationships that once offered comfort can become sources of frustration when that emotional 'switch' doesn't turn back on as it should.

Cognitively, the mind adapts to process information relentlessly, often focusing on adverse outcomes as a survival mechanism. This hyper-vigilance serves a soldier well when assessing threats but can lead to a tendency to anticipate danger where there is none, leading to anxiety and paranoia. The decision-making process in combat is often binary and immediate, which contrasts starkly with the nuanced and complex decisions required in civilian life, where choices come shaded in gray rather than the stark black and white of the battlefield.

The shift back to civilian life requires a retraining of emotional and cognitive responses—a task that can be daunting, to say the least. Veterans may struggle with irritability, impatience, or feelings of disconnection, compounded by a society that often misunderstands these challenges. Traditional therapies can offer strategies to manage these symptoms, yet some find these approaches lack the depth needed to reach the deeply ingrained patterns established in combat.

In exploring the potential of psychedelic-assisted psychotherapy, we delve into the ability of these substances to reach the emotional and cognitive roots planted in the field of battle. By carefully and responsibly harnessing their power, there is potential to revisit the emotional numbness and mental alertness of combat and reintegrate these experiences, recalibrating the emotional and cognitive dials. These therapies can offer a pathway to reawaken the spectrum of human feeling and thought, reconceptualize past experiences, and help veterans step fully and meaningfully into their present lives.

For those who have shielded their emotions and sharpened their minds to survive, this guide is an invitation to explore how psychedelic-assisted therapies might help veterans to thrive in a peacetime world that awaits their return.

Skillsets and Liabilities

The transformation from civilian to combatant is not merely a change in attire or environment but a fundamental reprogramming of the brain's approach to daily existence. Military training aims to instill skills that ensure survival and success in hostile environments and war. This training hones the mind to detect the faintest anomaly in a landscape, judge friend from foe instantly, and react with a speed that outpaces conscious thought. Situational awareness in combat zones is a skill and an all-consuming state where soldiers must be acutely attuned to their surroundings every waking moment.

For example, a soldier may develop an extraordinary ability to map environments quickly, recognizing safe routes and potential ambush points, a skill vital in combat chaos. In civilian life, however, this can translate to an exhausting hypervigilance that makes it impossible to relax even in safe environments. The rapid decision-making that can save lives on the battlefield might result in impulsivity at home, where decisions often benefit from reflection and consultation.

The constant readiness to engage with the enemy, to perceive a threat in every shadow, becomes an ingrained response. In civilian settings, this readiness does not fade away; it can manifest in startling reactions to benign stimuli, such as a veteran diving for cover at the sound of fireworks or feeling an irresistible urge to scan for exits and threats when entering a room.

This skillset also includes tactical thinking, the ability to strategize quickly and to adapt plans in real-time as situations evolve. It is a mindset of always being several steps ahead, anticipating and mitigating risks.

While advantageous in a theater of war, in civilian life, this can lead to an overwhelming sense of distrust and paranoia, where the veteran feels they must always be prepared for the worst-case scenario.

Furthermore, these deeply ingrained patterns of hyper-alertness and quick reaction times can intersect with sleep—another battlefield necessity that can become a peacetime affliction. Sleep in combat is often light and broken, a trait that allows an immediate response to threats but can evolve into full-blown insomnia when the perceived need for vigilance persists in a safe environment.

Understanding these transitions is crucial for both veterans and those who support them. Recognizing that what are now liabilities were once essential survival skills can provide a sense of empathy and context. It underscores the importance of retraining and adapting these skills to fit into a peaceful life—a process that requires time, patience, and often professional guidance.

Psychedelic-assisted psychotherapy can offer a unique approach to addressing these entrenched patterns. By inducing a state of altered consciousness, these therapies can facilitate a re-examination and re-integration of these combat-hardened skills, transforming them from liabilities into assets that enrich and enhance post-service life.

In this context, this guide seeks to offer a bridge between two worlds. It acknowledges the exceptional capabilities that soldiers bring back from combat and provides insights into how those capabilities can be reattributed. It's a roadmap for re-purposing the extraordinary war-forged skillsets for the benefit of the veteran, their families, and society at large.

The Continuum of Stress Responses

In understanding the continuum of stress responses, it's crucial to recognize that not all reactions to combat stress are pathological. Initially, many of these responses are ordinary and necessary adaptations to extreme environments. For instance, the quickened pulse, heightened alertness, and adrenaline rush are all part of the body's natural protective mechanisms. When these reactions don't subside after the threat has passed, they can become problematic.

Immediately following combat, it's common for veterans to experience a range of symptoms reflective of acute stress reactions. These can include jumpiness, irritability, difficulty concentrating, or sleep disturbances. Such symptoms are expected and are the mind and body's attempts to process and adapt to the intense experiences faced in combat. For many, given time and support, these symptoms gradually diminish.

However, some veterans find that the stress response becomes a chronic condition. The persistent state of being 'on alert' can lead to exhaustion and burnout. For example, a veteran may experience intrusive memories or flashbacks where it feels as though the combat experience is happening all over again. Sounds and sights can trigger these or even smells that resemble those of the battlefield, and they can be so vivid that they interfere with the ability to engage in everyday activities.

Moral injury is another critical aspect of the stress response continuum. This term refers to the distressing psychological, behavioral, emotional, and spiritual aftermath of exposure to events that go against an individual's moral or ethical code. A veteran might suffer from moral injury if they were involved in or witnessed actions that contradicted their values, such as harming civilians or failing to prevent such harm. This can lead to profound guilt, shame, and a loss of trust in oneself and others.

Substance use disorders often interplay with these stress responses, as alcohol or drugs may be used to self-medicate and alleviate the distress associated with them. While substance use might provide temporary relief, it can exacerbate symptoms in the long term, creating a detrimental cycle that can be hard to break.

To illustrate, a veteran might begin drinking or using substances to dull the edge of anxiety or to quiet the intrusive thoughts that plague them during sleep. Initially, it may seem like a viable way to cope, but over time, drinking can become a new battlefront as dependence grows, relationships strain, and health deteriorates.

The transition from acute stress responses to enduring mental health conditions underscores the need for timely and effective interventions. Early support and treatment can often prevent normal stress reactions from becoming chronic and debilitating conditions. In this light, the exploration of psychedelic-assisted psychotherapy presents a new frontier, offering hope for reprocessing traumatic memories, healing moral injuries, and addressing the root causes of substance use disorders.

This guide will delve into the complexities of these stress responses, examining the multifaceted nature of combat-related stress and the potential for psychedelic therapies to assist.

traditional methods may not have fully addressed the veteran's needs. It aims to illuminate the healing path, for the veterans and for the families and communities that are an integral part of their support network.

The Cultural and Spiritual Dimensions

The cultural and spiritual dimensions of a soldier's experience in combat are as diverse as the individuals who serve. Culture shapes the perception of duty, honor, and sacrifice, while spirituality offers a framework to understand the profound experiences of life and death. When the realities of war rattle the veil of belief, a veteran's underlying worldviews may be shaken, necessitating a search for new meaning or a reaffirmation of faith.

Culture provides a narrative for understanding the role of the warrior. Within this narrative, values are ascribed to actions and experiences. For instance, many Western cultures lionize the warrior archetype, associating it with bravery and heroism. However, when the lived experience of combat does not align with these heroic narratives, veterans can experience a dissonance between what they were culturally conditioned to expect and what they encountered. This clash can result in feelings of alienation, misunderstanding, and questioning one's cultural identity.

Conversely, some veterans return with a sense of cultural pride and fulfillment, feeling that they've embodied the values and virtues extolled by their society. These individuals often experience a smoother reintegration, bolstered by the alignment between their cultural expectations and personal experiences.

Spirituality often provides a context for the chaos of war, offering solace and a sense of purpose or destiny. The warrior may seek guidance from spiritual beliefs during moral conflict or after experiencing loss and tragedy. For some, there is a profound crisis of faith when the reality of war contradicts deeply held spiritual beliefs. Questions arise such as, "How could a just world allow such suffering?" or "Where is the divine in all this turmoil?"

For others, spirituality becomes a wellspring of resilience. Stories are plentiful of soldiers who, amid battle, found a deeper connection to their faith, a profound sense of being part of something larger than themselves. These experiences can lead to a strengthened spiritual identity and be integral to coping with the aftermath of combat.

Consider the story of devout Christian Sergeant Alvarez, who, upon returning from tours in Iraq, found himself lost, unable to reconcile the violence he'd seen with the pacifist principles of his upbringing. His journey through PTSD therapy focused on managing symptoms but but also enabled redefining his spiritual compass, finding peace with the past, and forging a new path that honored both his service and his core beliefs.

Then there's Captain Moore, for whom the principles of Buddhism provided a profound framework for understanding his experiences in combat and for reconciling his actions with his spiritual journey. The Buddhist teachings on karma and dharma, the ethical duty one carries out according to one's path in life, offered him a lens through which to view his service. The notion of "right action" within the Eightfold Path helped him to make peace with his experiences, framing them within the broader context of his commitment to alleviating suffering and upholding his duties as a soldier.

The inclusion of cultural and spiritual considerations in therapy is paramount. Traditional therapies may not fully address the depth of cultural dislocation or spiritual crisis that can occur after combat. This is where psychedelic-assisted psychotherapy could offer a unique avenue for exploration and healing by facilitating profound personal insights and spiritual experiences that can help veterans integrate their experiences in a way that aligns with their cultural and spiritual identities.

As we progress through this guide, we will explore how the intersection of culture, spirituality, and psychedelics can contribute to a holistic healing approach, offering a broader context for veterans as they navigate the challenging terrain of their post-combat lives.

The Return Home

The journey back from the battlefront is far more than a physical relocation; it is a passage through invisible barriers that separate the world of war from the world of those who await the warrior's return. For many veterans, transitioning from active duty to civilian life is not a homecoming but a foray into an entirely new battlefield with silent, unseen adversaries: memories, hypervigilance, and a pervasive sense of dislocation.

Take, for example, Sergeant Williams, who, upon returning from tours in Iraq, found himself in the cereal aisle of a grocery store, sweating and heart pounding, not from the threat of an IED, but from the overwhelming choices and the cacophony of everyday life—a stark contrast to the life-or-death simplicity of combat decisions. Or consider Specialist Ramirez, for whom a Fourth of July fireworks celebration became an ordeal of anxiety and flashbacks, the festive explosions indistinguishable from the sounds of mortar rounds.

These stories exemplify the latent echoes of war that intrude into the civilian life of a veteran. It's not merely about acclimating to life without uniforms and orders; it's about recalibrating the mind to not perceive threats in the benign, to not seek out the structure in the chaos of everyday living. For some, this reintegration process can take months; for others, it stretches into years or even a lifetime.

Moreover, the cultural gap between civilian and military life means that veterans often return to a society that may offer verbal thanks for their service but offer little tangible comprehension for the sacrifices made or the inner turmoil that service can entail. This gap can result in a profound sense of alienation. Veterans may feel they've come back to a home that no longer feels like home, where the language of their daily struggle is not spoken, and their experiences are relegated to the realm of the unfathomable.

The return home is thus not the end of the journey for a combat veteran; it is an ongoing process of finding a new equilibrium, a way to carry the weight of war within a peaceful context, to find meaning in a civilian existence that often seems trivial in comparison to the life-and-death clarity of combat. It is a silent march through a continuum of adjustment, showcasing the resilience and unyielding spirit of those who stood on the front lines.

The Family Dynamics

The homecoming of a combat veteran often carries with it an unspoken hope for restoration, a return to the familial roles and rhythms that preceded deployment. Yet, the family they return to is seldom the same as the one they left behind. The interlude of war reshapes a veteran in profound and sometimes imperceptible ways, even to themselves and their family. They must navigate these changes while grappling with the transformations that occurred during the absence.

Children who were infants when a parent deployed may now be walking and talking, partners may have taken on new roles and responsibilities, and parents may have aged or faced health issues. The dynamics that once seemed so natural now require conscious effort to renegotiate. For instance, a spouse may have become accustomed to making decisions independently and may currently struggle to reintegrate the veteran into family decision-making. Children might feel disconnected or intimidated by a parent who seems more stern or distant than they remember.

The psychological shifts experienced by the veteran can perplex and alarm family members. A father who once played with his children may now be irritable and withdrawn. A mother who easily juggles family life may now be overwhelmed by the noise and chaos of home. Sleep disturbances can fray tempers, and hypervigilance can cast a pall of tension over the household. Veterans might feel like outsiders in their homes, unable to reconnect with the intimacy and trust that once bound them to their loved ones.

Communication, essential to family cohesion, often becomes the most immediate casualty. Veterans might avoid discussing their experiences out of a desire to protect their families from the harsh realities of war or from a belief that they will not be understood. Families, in turn, may tiptoe around the veteran, unsure of how to bridge the widening emotional chasm.

As the veteran struggles with their internal turmoil, their family must confront a host of secondary stressors. They must learn to readjust expectations, communicate in new ways, and offer support while caring for their emotional well-being. It's a delicate balance of giving space while staying connected, providing support without enabling avoidance, and encouraging professional help while fostering mutual understanding and healing within the family unit.

In the complexity of reintegration, the family becomes both a sanctuary and a threat for the returning warrior. In this place, the war's invisible wounds are most acutely felt and where the most profound healing can occur. Within this intimate sphere, the work of reintegration unfolds, requiring patience, compassion, and, often, the assistance of outside support to guide the way.

The impact of combat, with its profound and pervasive influence, creates a complex narrative within the warrior's psyche and, by extension, within their community. It's an enduring narrative that shapes their physical responses, molds their emotional contours, and defines their cognitive outlook. This narrative belongs to veterans and their closest allies— family, friends, and fellow service members.

As we conclude this chapter, we have cultivated a minute understanding of the multifaceted nature of combat and its long-lasting effects on those who endure it. This understanding is crucial as we address the aftermath of such service, particularly the numerous mental health challenges that arise.

In the chapters that follow, we will explore a spectrum of therapeutic modalities, with a keen focus on the promising and potent role of psychedelic-assisted therapies. These therapies are significant offering innovative avenues for addressing deep-seated psychological wounds. We approach these modalities cautiously and optimistically, acknowledging their potential as catalysts for profound transformation and healing.

With the groundwork laid, our journey ahead will illuminate the healing pathways for our veterans. By integrating the wisdom of conventional therapies with the transformative potential of psychedelics, we strive to open doors to newfound well-being, guiding our warriors and their families toward a future where peace of mind and spirit can be reclaimed.

CHAPTER 2

Aftermath of Combat: PTSD, Moral Injury, Reintegration, and Other Mental Health Challenges

As the echoes of battle fade into a haunting silence for many combat veterans, the unspoken tremors of war reverberate through the mind and soul, manifesting as the invisible wounds of post-traumatic stress disorder (PTSD) and moral injury. The healing journey is as personal as the memories that linger; it beckons a multifaceted approach that honors the complexity of the human spirit. Amongst these healing modalities, psychedelic-assisted psychotherapy emerges as a beacon of hope, casting new light on the shadows that many warriors carry within.

Psychedelic-assisted psychotherapy, a field combining the profound insights of psychology with the altered states of consciousness induced by psychedelics, has shown promise in recent empirical research. The therapeutic context is paramount; it is not merely about the substance but the synergistic dance between the medicine, the mind, and the skilled guidance of a therapist. This dance can catalyze profound trans-formations, often described by veterans as a reawakening to life.

Through a lens that integrates the medical, psychological, and metaphysical, we explore how psychedelics, within a therapeutic framework, may assist combat veterans in renegotiating the terms of their inner battles. Informed by Eastern and Western philosophies, this chapter aims to distill wisdom as ancient as the Vedas and as modern as the latest neuroscience.

As you journey through this chapter, allow the provocative nature of this subject to challenge your perceptions and the detailed discourse to offer new insights. The emotional tone is set to be empathetic, recognizing the courage it takes to confront one's vulnerabilities. Let this introduction serve not only to inform but to inspire a quest for deeper understanding and healing; and, as we delve into the complexities of the mind and the potential of psychedelics to unlock healing, we do so with the utmost respect for the individuals who have donned the uniform in service to others.

Finally, while the promise of psychedelic-assisted psychotherapy shines bright, it is essential to acknowledge the necessity of professional guidance. This chapter underscores the importance of seeking skilled therapists who can navigate the delicate realms of the psyche with veterans, ensuring a safe and transformative experience.

In the following chapters, 'The Silent Echoes of Battle' will unfold, revealing the intricacies of the inner war that many veterans face and the emerging modalities that offer hope and healing.

The Silent Echoes of Battle

The battlefield may lie silent, yet within many combat veterans, the war rages on. This internal conflict, known as Post-Traumatic Stress Disorder (PTSD), is a psychological scar, a reaction to the unbearable stressors that soldiers often encounter. PTSD is more than a list of symptoms; it represents a profound disruption of a person's core being, their sense of safety, and their trust in the world.

Through the Lens of Combat Experience, PTSD is not merely a psychiatric condition but a profoundly personal, all-encompassing response to the horrific experiences of war. The high incidence of PTSD among veterans can be attributed to the intensity and frequency of combat exposure, which dramatically escalates the risk of developing this condition (Peterson et al., 2011). War, in its most visceral form, presents scenarios that are beyond the realm of everyday human experience—exposure to death, severe injury, and the moral injuries that come with combat. Such experiences can deeply impact the psyche, often resulting in symptoms that persist long after the individual has left the battlefield.

The Diagnostic and Statistical Manual of Mental Disorders (DSM-5) outlines specific criteria for diagnosing PTSD, a structured approach that helps to quantify and address the subjective experiences of veterans. The criteria encompass a wide range of symptoms, from the re-experiencing of traumatic events (Criterion B), such as flashbacks and nightmares, to behavioral changes like avoidance (Criterion C), negative alterations in cognition and mood (Criterion D), and alterations in arousal and reactivity (Criterion E). The DSM-5 emphasizes that these symptoms must cause significant impairment in personal, social, or occupational domains (Criterion G) and are not attributable to other factors (Criterion H).

The Multidimensional Nature of PTSD in combat veterans is distinguished by its direct tie to life-threatening events specific to the battlefield. This connection is crucial because it underscores the multifaceted nature of the disorder, involving the mind and the entire being of a person. As outlined by the American Psychiatric Association (2013), a significant portion of combat-exposed veterans may meet the criteria for PTSD, pointing to the urgent need for effective interventions.

PTSD is often associated with vivid, intrusive re-experiences of combat, including nightmares and flashbacks, which can disrupt a veteran's day-to-day life (APA, 2013). These are not mere memories but visceral re-livings of the trauma, so intense that the veteran may feel as though they are back on the battlefield. Avoidant behaviors are another hallmark of PTSD, where veterans may steer clear of situations or thoughts that remind them of their traumatic experiences. This can lead to a narrowing of their lives and can impede the healing process. Moreover, the constant state of heightened alertness and the changes in cognition and mood can strain relationships, making feelings of isolation and detachment all too common among veterans with PTSD.

Integrating empirical research and therapeutic approaches is vital in understanding the neurobiological and psychological underpinnings of PTSD. Studies have shown changes in the brain, such as alterations in the amygdala and prefrontal cortex, which are associated with processing fear and regulating emotions (Shin et al., 2006). Such insights are invaluable as they pave the way for developing targeted therapies to address these changes.

Addressing PTSD in the context of psychedelic-assisted psychotherapy offers a novel approach to treating PTSD by combining psychotherapeutic techniques with the administration of psychedelics. Emerging research suggests that psychedelics can facilitate neuroplasticity, fostering new patterns of thought and behavior that can be transformative for individuals who have PTSD. This therapy's empathetic and grounded approach aligns with the need for veterans to be understood and supported through their healing process.

When discussing psychedelic-assisted psychotherapy, a compelling narrative emerges. It's a narrative that not only reflects the stark reality of PTSD but also the potential for recovery and growth. Research suggests that with proper guidance and a safe, supportive environment, veterans can begin to confront their trauma, engaging with their memories and experiences in a way that fosters healing rather than avoidance.

Understanding PTSD in combat veterans requires a comprehensive view that appreciates the depth of combat's impact on the human psyche. It is a condition that necessitates interventions as rigorous as they are compassionate. Psychedelic-assisted psychotherapy, with its empirical grounding and multidisciplinary approach, presents a promising avenue for helping veterans reclaim a sense of peace and purpose.

Moral Injury and Inner Conflict: The Wounds Beyond the Battlefield

In the quest to reconcile the realm of war's reality with the inner sanctum of personal ethics, combat veterans often grapple with moral injury—a profound psychological scar marked by an agonizing moral paradox. It's not simply the recollection of life-threatening events that haunts them, as in PTSD, but the violation of their moral compass, which inflicts a unique form of suffering.

Moral injury, in its essence, is the profound psychological distress that arises when a person perpetrates, fails to prevent, bears witness to, or learns about acts that transgress their deeply held moral beliefs and expectations. For combat veterans, these are not mere abstractions, but visceral experiences etched into their souls through the unfathomable realities of war.

The statistics are harrowing. Over half of war-exposed combatants have been in situations where they have directed lethal force toward others; many have been the instruments of mortality themselves. The sight of human remains and the haunting experiences of not being able to assist the wounded or innocent, especially children, sear into their consciousness. Nearly all report participation or witness to acts they deem morally reprehensible, sowing seeds of biopsychosocial turmoil.

This internal dissonance can unleash a cascade of psychological upheavals, often precipitating guilt, shame, and self-condemnation. These emotions, if unaddressed, may gnaw at the very essence of one's identity, precipitating a host of adverse outcomes, including severe psychological distress and even suicidal ideation.

It is crucial to discern that while moral injury and PTSD may share a common genesis in the traumatic construct of combat, they are distinct entities. PTSD is grounded in the fear for one's life; moral injury, by contrast, stems from the confrontation with ethical transgressions—actions that irrevocably conflict with one's sense of right and wrong. They may intersect and influence each other, with moral injury often predicting the re-experiencing and avoidance symptoms seen in PTSD. Yet, they do not equate to the same diagnostic criteria.

This distinction is paramount in the therapeutic arena. While PTSD is a recognized psychiatric disorder, moral injury is not yet formally classified as such. However, its impact on a veteran's ability to function —in the family, at work, and within society—can be equally, if not more, debilitating. Clinicians must identify and distinguish these experiences, as the therapeutic strategies to address them may differ significantly. The treatment of moral injury must go beyond the clinical and delve into the moral and spiritual domains, requiring a holistic approach that integrates principles from both Eastern and Western thought. This may include mindfulness and compassion-based interventions, narrative therapy, and practices encouraging the veteran's reintegration into a moral community.

Understanding the depth and breadth of moral injury is a clarion call for a more nuanced and compassionate response to the unseen wounds of war. This understanding is the first step toward healing and wholeness for the veteran, their families, and the clinicians who serve them.

Reintegration Challenges

The transition from active military duty back to civilian life marks a critical phase in the lives of combat veterans—a journey often beset with reintegration challenges. This complex metamorphosis entails personal transformation and restructuring roles within family, community, and the workplace. Such a multilayered transition involves a dynamic interplay between the individual veteran and the societal framework awaiting their return.

At the heart of reintegration issues is an identity crisis, a profound struggle as veterans seek to reconcile the stark dichotomy between military and civilian cultures. The military instills a distinctive warrior identity that might not seamlessly align with civilian life. This identity, often shaped by the necessity of life-or-death decision-making and exposure to the horrors of combat, may become a source of inner conflict as veterans leave the structured environment of the armed forces. In some cases, veterans grapple with the residues of moral injury, a form of psychological stress resulting from actions that violate one's ethical code. Such distress can lead to self-identity disintegration, fostering isolation and a sense of alienation within the broader social fabric.

Veterans facing reintegration challenges frequently exhibit higher incidences of mental health disorders such as PTSD and depression. These conditions can significantly hinder a veteran's ability to function effectively in social, familial, and occupational spheres. Mental illness can strain family dynamics, complicate the transition to civilian employment, and compound the veteran's distress. The ramification of these challenges is a comprehensive social issue that demands a multifaceted and empathetic approach.

Addressing these reintegration challenges necessitates a holistic strategy that embraces the veteran's personal experiences and the broader ecological context of their lives. Support systems need to be tuned to the psychological aspects of the transition and the cultural, familial, and occupational domains that are integral to the veteran's new role in civilian life. This calls for a concerted effort from mental health professionals, community leaders, and policymakers to facilitate a smoother reintegration process for our veterans, ensuring that the transition from the battlefield to the home front is met with understanding, support, and honor.

The Mental Health Frontline: Depression, Anxiety, Substance Use, Homelessness, and Suicide. The battlefield is not the only place where veterans encounter life-altering challenges; the return to civilian life can bring its own frontline of mental health battles. It is essential to recognize that beyond the familiar territory of Post-Traumatic Stress Disorder (PTSD) and moral injury, a myriad of mental health issues can besiege veterans, such as depression, anxiety, substance use, homelessness, and the ultimate tragedy—suicide.

Depression looms as a particularly insidious foe. It is the most diagnosed mental health condition among returning veterans, surpassing even PTSD. With 23% of active-duty members and roughly 20% of all veterans diagnosed with Major Depressive Disorder, the scale of the affliction is vast, impacting a tremendous number of Americans serving and back in civilian life. This prevalence of depression, often chronic and co-existing with PTSD and Substance Use Disorder, diminishes the quality of life and, without adequate treatment, can escalate to life-threatening despair.

Anxiety disorders, encompassing Generalized Anxiety Disorder, Panic Disorder, and Social Anxiety Disorder, are characterized by pervasive worry and irrational fears that impede everyday functioning. Within the veteran population, research indicates that 18% of those seeking care at VA Health Clinics are diagnosed with an anxiety disorder, and a staggering 75% report symptoms of anxiety. This prevalence underscores the enduring nature of such conditions, which often persist alongside PTSD, leading to severe societal and personal hardships.

Substance Use Disorders are notably prevalent among veterans, with post-2011 veterans showing a significant propensity to these struggles. The link between combat exposure, PTSD, and substance use is well-documented, with over 20% of veterans with PTSD also grappling with substance use disorders—often manifesting as binge drinking behaviors.

The presence of veterans starkly marks the landscape of homelessness in the United States. A significant portion of the homeless population has served in the armed forces; in fact, a survey by the National Coalition for Homeless Veterans reveals a troubling statistic: 23 percent of all homeless persons and 33 percent of all homeless men are veterans. This suggests that between 529,000 and 840,000 veterans experience homelessness at some point during any given year.

Veterans face a disproportionately high risk of homelessness compared to their civilian counterparts. Factors contributing to this elevated risk include the prevalence of mental health issues and substance use disorders, the impact of PTSD, and the transition stress from military to civilian life. Moreover, veterans comprise roughly one in seven of all adults experiencing homelessness, with a significant number at risk of homelessness due to economic and mental health challenges. On a single night in January 2012, over 67,000 unsheltered veterans were found living on the streets, underscoring the urgent need for effective interventions and support.

The plight of homeless veterans is exacerbated by their higher rates of psychological and medical issues relative to the general homeless population, alongside substantial barriers to accessing care. As the Veterans Administration offers many services and treatments, the critical step is connecting those veterans in need to these resources. Despite availability, as Hoge et al. (2014) highlight, many veterans in need do not seek out VA facilities for support, suggesting a gap in outreach and engagement that must be addressed to mitigate the issue of veteran homelessness.

Despite the availability of treatment and services through the Veterans Administration, there is a concerning trend of veterans not seeking the help they require. Whether due to stigma, lack of awareness, or barriers to access, this gap between need and treatment is a chasm that must be bridged.

The escalation of mental health diagnoses among veterans since the commencement of the war on terror is a call to action. Mental illness is not merely a risk factor for challenges such as homelessness—it is often a determinant. Recognizing these conditions, understanding their interplay, and responding with the same strategic precision used in military operations is imperative in the quest to provide our veterans with the support and care they deserve.

Toward Healing: Psychotherapy and Beyond

Acknowledging the scars is merely the first step. The actual journey begins with the first steps on the healing path. The principles of psychotherapy provide a solid foundation, yet there is an emerging dialogue around the role of psychedelics in this space. Meticulously researched and responsibly approached, psychedelic-assisted psychotherapy offers a potential adjunct to traditional methods, weaving together the threads of medical, psychological, and spiritual approaches to forge a new path to wellness.

The synthesis of psychedelics and psychotherapy emerges not as a panacea but as a promising tool that deserves careful consideration. The anecdotes of the authors retreat experiences, coupled with his military and therapeutic expertise, shed light on the transformative potential of these substances when integrated into a holistic treatment plan. This discussion remains grounded in rigorous science and is punctuated with real-world insights, aiming to demystify and contextualize this ground-breaking approach for combat veterans and their families.

Healing is not a journey taken alone. Recovery is interwoven with the threads of community support and collective understanding. We expand the conversation to include the role of leadership, community engagement, and the power of shared experiences in healing.

In this multi-part exploration of the post-combat landscape, the aim is to provide clarity and depth, challenging readers to engage with difficult questions and explore the full scope of mental health challenges faced by combat veterans. With an empathetic and scholarly tone, the goal is to encourage, inspire, and ultimately illuminate the path forward.

CHAPTER 3

Conventional & Alternative Therapies

Combat veterans confront a gauntlet of psychological adversities upon reintegration into civilian life, adversities that are often compounded by barriers to accessing care. Traditional therapeutic interventions—comprising mainly pharmaceuticals and structured psychotherapies—offer a lifeline for many. However, there's a staggering discrepancy between the availability of these treatments and the veterans' willingness or ability to seek them out. Veterans may wait years, sometimes decades, before pursuing help for mental health issues. According to a report by the Substance Abuse and Mental Health Services Administration (SAMHSA), the average time from military discharge to seeking care can be as long as 12.7 years for veterans with PTSD.

The reluctance to seek care is multifaceted. Stigma, pride, and a pervasive culture of self-reliance are often significant hindrances. This aversion to seeking help is illustrated in a sobering statistic from the Department of Veterans Affairs, which estimates that only 50% of returning veterans who need mental health treatment will receive these services.

When veterans do seek care, the quality of counseling can vary dramatically. Effective counseling requires an in-depth understanding of general psychological principles and an acute sensitivity to the specific

experiences and cultural nuances of the military and veteran populations. Unfortunately, mental health professionals are not adequately
trained in these areas. A 2015 RAND study found that only 13% of
U.S. mental health providers met the criteria for military cultural competency, which encompasses an understanding of military ethos, the
distinctive aspects of the combat experience, and the ramifications of
military service on mental health.

Furthermore, veterans often report a disconnect when counselors,
albeit well-intentioned, lack direct experience with military culture or
combat. This gap can contribute to ineffective therapeutic alliances,
hindering treatment and outcomes. In some instances, this deficiency in
training and understanding may not only render the therapy ineffective
but could exacerbate the veterans' conditions by reinforcing feelings of
isolation and being misunderstood.

Effective counseling is also impeded by systemic challenges, such
as bureaucracy within veteran services and limited access to care, particularly in rural areas. While efforts have been made to address these
challenges, such as through the Veterans Choice Program, which allows
veterans to receive care from community providers, there remains much
work to be done to ensure all veterans have timely access to competent,
empathetic, and effective mental health care.

These complexities underscore a vital need for a comprehensive over-
haul of the support system available to combat veterans. This system
not only makes therapeutic services available but also ensures these services are adequately tailored to address the deeply individual and often
complex needs of those who have served. As we move forward, it is crucial to consider alternative therapeutic modalities, such as psychedelic-
assisted psychotherapy, which may offer more holistic and potentially
productive avenues for healing the psychological wounds of war.

Pharmaceutical Interventions

In the therapeutic arsenal for combat-related psychological conditions, pharmaceutical treatments frequently form the vanguard.

Antidepressants, anxiolytics, benzodiazepines, mood stabilizers, and other psychotropic medications are commonly prescribed to manage the symptoms of post-traumatic stress disorder (PTSD), depression, anxiety, and other mental health issues that veterans face. These medications can function as critical stabilizers, reducing the acuteness of symptoms and potentially granting veterans the necessary reprieve to engage in other forms of therapy.

However, the application of these pharmaceuticals has significant caveats. Principally, while they can mitigate symptoms, they seldom address the underlying psychological traumas that trigger these symptoms. Their relief is symptomatic and often surface-level, leaving the root causes of distress unexplored and unprocessed. This limitation can result in a state of perpetual medication reliance, with little progress resolving core issues.

The quandary of overmedication among veterans is a critical concern, manifesting in the excessive use of prescribed medications, particularly opioids, which are often given for chronic pain—a common affliction in this population. The Department of Veterans Affairs has reported high rates of opioid prescription among veterans, which intersects alarmingly with mental health disorders, heightening the risk for substance misuse and overdose.

The side effects of psychotropic medications add another layer of complexity to an already challenging situation. These can range from mild discomforts such as headaches and nausea to severe impacts on physical and mental health, including increased suicidal ideation, a paradoxical increase in anxiety, weight gain, and sexual dysfunction. The aggregate of these side effects can severely diminish the quality of life and may even exacerbate a veteran's sense of disconnection from self and society.

Dependency is another grave concern. Some veterans may develop a psychological or physiological dependence on these medications, especially benzodiazepines and opioids. This often leads to a long-term cycle where the medication becomes a crutch rather than a cure. In the context of combat veterans, who often endure a matrix of physical and emotional scars, the risk of dependency poses a significant challenge to achieving genuine and sustained mental health.

It is incumbent upon healthcare providers and support systems to recognize that while pharmacotherapy can play a role in managing symptoms, it should be integrated with a broader, more holistic approach to mental health. Such an approach would consider the individual's entire biopsychosocial experience and include therapies aimed at processing trauma, building resilience, and fostering growth beyond symptom management. Only by acknowledging and addressing the multifaceted nature of a veteran's healing journey can we begin to move beyond the paradigm of overmedication.

Psychotherapeutic Interventions

Cognitive Behavioral Therapy (CBT) stands as a cornerstone within the therapeutic community for its structured, evidence-based approach to treating psychological disorders. A meta-analysis of CBT for PTSD, for instance, suggests moderate efficacy, with a sizeable proportion of patients experiencing significant symptom reduction. Studies consistently show that CBT can lead to a decrease in symptoms of anxiety and depression, with roughly 50-60% of patients with these disorders deriving benefit from this modality.

The crux of CBT lies in its ability to help individuals recognize and reframe maladaptive thought patterns, fostering a more adaptive and constructive engagement with their thoughts and feelings. This reframing process is rooted in enhancing cognitive skills to dismantle the automatic negative thought cycles that can govern emotional well-being.

Yet, despite its widespread application and success, CBT's efficacy is not uniformly felt across all populations. Veterans grappling with complex trauma present a particular challenge to the CBT paradigm. Combat-related trauma often transcends the cognitive dimension, engrained not only in the mind but also in the bodily experience of the individual. It can manifest as an intricate co-occurrence of grief, guilt, and moral injury, interlaced with the veteran's identity and perception of the world.

A certain level of cognitive functioning is requisite for CBT to be effective, particularly within the prefrontal cortex, which governs reasoning, planning, and problem-solving processes. However, individuals who are severely dysregulated due to PTSD or those suffering from a traumatic brain injury (TBI) may find it challenging to engage with the cognitive and cerebral demands of CBT. This dysregulation can impair the executive functions necessary to benefit from CBT's more structured tasks and reflective exercises.

Moreover, when it comes to the processing of trauma, CBT might provide less opportunity for individuals to engage with and process their experiences on a sensory and emotional level, which can be essential for those whose traumatic experiences are stored in non-verbal, sensory memories. The very nature of PTSD can make it challenging for sufferers to access and articulate their thoughts and feelings—a prerequisite for CBT's effectiveness.

It is, therefore, vital for therapists to evaluate the cognitive readiness of their clients before engaging in CBT. Alternative or adjunct therapies, such as sensorimotor psychotherapy or Eye Movement Desensitization and Reprocessing (EMDR), which do not rely as heavily on verbal processing and cognitive reframing, may be more suitable for those with cognitive limitations or those who find CBT's approach too challenging at the outset of treatment.

While CBT is a potent tool for many psychological disorders, its applicability and efficacy in treating combat veterans must be considered with nuance. It is essential to ensure that the individual veteran has the cognitive capacity and is in a sufficiently regulated state to engage with the therapy effectively. For those who do not meet these criteria, alternative treatments should be explored that can meet the veterans where they are in their healing journey.

Mindfulness, with its origins in ancient contemplative traditions, has traversed a long historical pathway to become a component of modern psychotherapeutic practices. Its use in psychological contexts is supported by a wealth of empirical evidence accumulated over the past few decades. Research, including randomized control trials and neuro-biological studies, has indicated that mindfulness practices can significantly reduce symptoms of depression, anxiety, and post-traumatic stress disorder (PTSD), contributing to an overall enhancement in the quality of life.

At the core of mindfulness is the cultivation of a present-focused, non-judgmental awareness. By adopting this stance, individuals learn to observe their thoughts and feelings as transient mental events rather than as defining aspects of their identity or experiences. This shift can profoundly alter the relationship to traumatic memories and sensations, creating a space for healing and growth.

The effectiveness of mindfulness is grounded in its ability to engage the brain's present-moment pathway, fostering a sense of calm and focus that can contrast sharply with the chaotic and intrusive thoughts characteristic of PTSD and other stress-related disorders. Mindfulness can help recalibrate the nervous system, promoting self-regulation and resilience. Moreover, psychoeducation—the process of educating individuals about psychological concepts—enhances mindfulness by demystifying mental health issues and empowering individuals with knowledge and self-care strategies.

Despite its effectiveness and longstanding history, mindfulness is not without its limitations, especially when considering the unique challenges faced by combat veterans with PTSD or traumatic brain injury (TBI). The dysregulation mindfulness seeks to ease can also present a significant barrier to its successful implementation. For individuals in the throes of PTSD or those who have sustained TBIs, achieving the level of focus necessary to engage in mindfulness practices can be daunting. Symptoms such as hypervigilance, flashbacks, and cognitive impairments can impede the capacity to maintain the sustained attention and awareness that mindfulness requires.

Additionally, medications commonly prescribed for PTSD and other trauma-related symptoms can sometimes interfere with cognitive processes. Certain psychotropic drugs may dampen emotional responses and cognitive alertness, which can paradoxically hinder the full activation of the present-moment awareness that mindfulness aims to foster.

Therefore, it is essential to approach mindfulness as one tool within a comprehensive therapeutic toolkit tailored to each veteran's unique circumstances. For those struggling with significant dysregulation, mindfulness practices may need to be adapted or introduced gradually, often in concert with other therapeutic interventions that prioritize stabilization and safety. Similarly, psychoeducation can play a critical role in setting realistic expectations and providing a roadmap for integrating mindfulness into everyday life, even amid challenges.

Mindfulness and psychoeducation collectively offer a promising avenue for addressing the scars of combat, but they must be delivered with an understanding of their limitations. Therapists and practitioners must recognize the nuanced ways in which dysregulation and medication can impact the therapeutic process and be prepared to adjust their approach accordingly to accommodate the diverse needs of veterans navigating the path to recovery.

Exposure therapies, particularly prolonged exposure therapy (PE) and cognitive processing therapy (CPT) represent a cornerstone in the treatment of PTSD, drawing upon principles of cognitive-behavioral therapy. These methods are grounded in the belief that therapeutic confrontation with traumatic memories is essential for processing and integration, ultimately leading to symptom reduction.

PE therapy encourages individuals to gradually revisit and recount their traumatic experiences in a safe and controlled environment, aiming to reduce fear and avoidance behaviors. CPT, on the other hand, focuses on identifying and challenging maladaptive beliefs related to trauma, facilitating cognitive restructuring, and the development of a new understanding of the traumatic event.

The empirical support for exposure therapies is robust, with numerous studies documenting their efficacy. Success rates for PE and CPT are cited to be high, with many individuals experiencing a significant decrease in the intensity and frequency of PTSD symptoms.

However, despite their healing potential, these therapies are not without risks. The intensity of revisiting traumatic events can be profound, and without the appropriate support and coping mechanisms in place, there is a risk of re-traumatization. The dropout rates for exposure therapies can be significant, as the distress elicited can sometimes feel overwhelming for veterans, leading them to discontinue therapy prematurely. Secondary traumatization—the emotional duress that results when an individual is exposed to the firsthand trauma experiences of others—is also a risk, particularly for therapists or family members involved in the therapeutic process.

Veterans who engage in these therapies need careful preparation, monitoring, and follow-up to ensure that the process is manageable. Therapists must be skilled not only in the delivery of these therapeutic modalities but also in the detection of signs of increased distress and the application of stabilization techniques when necessary. Therapeutic sessions should be paced according to the individual's capacity to process traumatic content without becoming overwhelmed.

It's important to acknowledge that not all veterans are suitable candidates for exposure therapies, especially those with complex PTSD, severe dissociation, or comorbid conditions such as substance use disorders. In such cases, other treatment options or preliminary stabilizing interventions may be necessary before exposure therapies can be considered.

Exposure therapies are a powerful tool in the arsenal against PTSD, but they must be applied with precision, compassion, and sensitivity to the veteran's psychological state. By carefully managing these therapies and individualizing treatment plans, practitioners can help veterans navigate the difficult terrain of their traumatic memories, turning a path of potential re-traumatization into one of recovery and growth.

Eye Movement Desensitization and Reprocessing (EMDR) stands as one of the more innovative and controversial treatments in the therapeutic armamentarium for trauma. It's a form of psychotherapy that has been extensively researched and has gained recognition for its effectiveness, especially in the treatment of PTSD.

The core mechanism of EMDR involves the patient recalling distressing images while receiving one of several types of bilateral sensory input, such as side-to-side eye movements or hand tapping. This process may facilitate the accessing and processing of traumatic memories, potentially allowing for a reorganization of these memories so they are no longer debilitating.

EMDR has shown promise in the rapid amelioration of distressing symptoms. The American Psychological Association (APA) recognizes it as effective for treating symptoms of acute and chronic PTSD. For veterans, who often carry a heavy burden of such memories, the potential relief EMDR promises is significant.

However, EMDR's effectiveness is not uniform across all individuals. The response to treatment can be highly variable, and this is particularly true for combat veterans, whose experiences often involve repeated and complex traumas. There are hypotheses that this variability may be due to differences in individual trauma histories, comorbid conditions, and personal resiliency.

Moreover, there's an ongoing debate within the psychological community regarding how EMDR works. Some suggest the effectiveness of EMDR may come from its similarities with other forms of therapy, such as the therapeutic relationship and elements of exposure therapy, rather than from the eye movement component itself.

Despite these discussions, EMDR is considered relatively low-risk and can be a valuable part of a comprehensive treatment plan, especially when tailored to the individual's needs and delivered by a trained professional. The Department of Veterans Affairs has incorporated EMDR into its treatment guidelines, indicating its perceived value in treating veterans with PTSD.

As with all treatments, it is essential to conduct thorough assessments prior to EMDR to ensure that it is an appropriate treatment modality for the individual veteran. For those who engage in EMDR therapy, the provision of a supportive and empathetic therapeutic environment is critical to foster the best outcomes. With continued research and clinical refinement, EMDR may increasingly be seen as a core element of effective interventions for combat-related trauma.

Virtual Reality Exposure Therapy (VRET) represents a cutting-edge convergence of technology and therapeutic techniques. It utilizes immersive virtual environments to safely expose individuals to the situations related to their traumatic experiences without the risks associated with real-life exposure. This controlled, gradual approach to exposure therapy allows veterans to confront and process trauma-related emotions and memories in a secure and supportive setting.

The principle behind VRET is akin to traditional exposure therapy: by repeatedly confronting the feared object, situation, or memory in a safe environment, the individual can learn to reduce their fear response. However, VRET's advantage lies in its ability to create a vivid yet controllable, multisensory experience that can be more engaging and less threatening than imagining a traumatic event. This can increase the veteran's sense of presence and emotional engagement during therapy without overwhelming them.

Preliminary research indicates that VRET can be effective for combat-related PTSD. It may reduce avoidance behaviors and improve symptoms of hyperarousal by allowing veterans to face their traumas in a way that traditional talk therapy cannot replicate. It's important to note that the efficacy of VRET can depend on the individual's response to virtual environments and the quality of the virtual reality content itself.

Complementing such technology-based approaches are psychosocial rehabilitation programs that focus on improving veterans' social and occupational functioning. These programs offer workshops, social skills training, job coaching, and community reintegration activities, providing a scaffold to rebuild a life post-service. However, they often fall short of providing in-depth psychological support, which is crucial for veterans grappling with severe mental health issues. These initiatives may inadvertently overlook the profound psychological wounds that require more than skill-building and knowledge to heal.

Both VRET and psychosocial rehabilitation are parts of the larger spectrum of veteran care, addressing different needs in the continuum of healing. While promising, they must be integrated with comprehensive mental health care and, ideally, personalized to each veteran's unique circumstances. The effective application of these innovative interventions requires a collaborative effort among healthcare providers, mental health professionals, and support systems. Only through such integration can the full potential of these approaches be realized in aiding veterans to process their experiences and transition to civilian life successfully.

Alternative Therapeutic Options

Experiential therapies, such as wilderness therapy and adventure-based counseling, offer veterans a departure from clinical settings, tapping into the healing powers of nature and physical activity. Such therapies can lead to improvements in self-esteem, provide a sense of accomplishment, and foster peer support. Despite these benefits, research on their long-term efficacy is still emerging, and they may not be as accessible for all veterans due to geographic or physical limitations.

Equine therapy, which involves interacting with horses, has shown promise for individuals with PTSD by promoting emotional growth and personal insight. The non-verbal communication and the bond formed with the animal can help veterans develop new ways to handle stress and relate to others. However, its efficacy varies, and it may not appeal to everyone, particularly those with certain physical disabilities or those who are uncomfortable around animals.

Light therapy, primarily used to treat seasonal affective disorder, has also been considered for PTSD to regulate sleep-wake cycles and improve mood. While its application for combat-related PTSD requires further research, it offers a low-risk option that could potentially benefit those with sleep disturbances related to their mental health conditions.

Both acupuncture and acupressure have been utilized for their stress-reducing and pain-relieving effects. For veterans, these practices can offer a non-pharmaceutical option to manage symptoms of PTSD and associated pain conditions. The evidence supporting their use is promising, yet it's important to note that qualified professionals should deliver such treatments to ensure safety and efficacy.

Other alternative treatments gaining attention include yoga, meditation, and art therapy. These practices emphasize mindfulness and self-expression, providing veterans with tools to manage stress and emotional dysregulation. The body-mind connection these disciplines foster can be particularly helpful in regaining a sense of control and peace. However, they may only resonate with some individuals, and their effectiveness can be influenced by a veteran's openness to these practices.

While non-traditional and alternative treatments offer valuable options for veterans seeking healing from combat-related traumas, they should not be viewed as standalone solutions. Their efficacy can be enhanced when integrated into a comprehensive treatment plan that is tailored to the individual needs of the veteran. Healthcare providers need to consider these options within the broader context of a multidisciplinary approach that accounts for the diverse preferences and experiences of combat veterans.

***

The landscape of current treatments for combat veterans often presents as a patchwork— effective in parts but lacking a unifying thread that addresses the multifaceted nature of military trauma. The limitations of these treatments often stem from a narrow scope that fails to encompass the collective dimensions of healing and underestimates the impact of cultural factors on treatment engagement. Many highly skilled and experienced clinicians are incorporating an eclectic multidimensional approach, implementing various strategies simultaneously. This multidimensional approach does show a slightly increased efficacy but is also encumbered with the same limitations as discussed.

One critical issue is the cultural context of military service, which is steeped in values such as strength, resilience, and self-reliance. These values can foster a sense of ambivalence or outright resistance for acknowledging psychological distress and seeking help. Stigmatization of mental health issues within military communities often exacerbates this problem, leading to underutilization of available treatments. The machismo culture can particularly deter veterans from expressing vulnerabilities and can be an obstacle to engaging with therapies that require emotional openness.

Additionally, there is a profound sense of moral injury that is frequently encountered by combat veterans. Moral injury arises from actions or witnessed events that transgress deeply held moral beliefs and expectations. Current treatment modalities like CBT or pharmaceutical interventions may not adequately address the complex existential and ethical distress that comes with moral injury. The inability of these treatments to tend to the moral and spiritual dimensions of combat experiences can leave veterans feeling isolated and misunderstood.

Furthermore, conventional therapies often operate within an individualistic framework, which may not align with the communal and collective experiences that veterans identify with. Healing, from many cultural and philosophical perspectives, is not solely an individual journey but a collective passage where community support and shared understanding play pivotal roles. This disconnect can lead to treatments that feel alienating or irrelevant to veterans accustomed to the camaraderie and brotherhood/sisterhood of military life.

Considering these limitations, there is a growing need to broaden the therapeutic options available to combat veterans. Approaches that incorporate community support, address moral and spiritual concerns, and combat stigma are essential. Integrating these elements into treatment could foster a more hospitable environment for veterans to seek care and adhere to therapies, ultimately improving outcomes.

As we delve deeper into the potential of psychedelic-assisted psychotherapy in subsequent chapters, we will explore how these treatments may offer a more holistic approach, one that resonates with the values and experiences of combat veterans and addresses the communal aspects of healing that are often missing in conventional therapies.

As we navigate the complexities of treating combat-related mental health issues, we recognize the courage of those who have served and the need for an integrated, multifaceted approach to healing. In the following chapters, we will delve into how psychedelic-assisted psychotherapy might fill the gaps left by conventional treatments, offering new hope and paths to recovery for combat veterans and their families.

PART II

Understanding Psychedelics

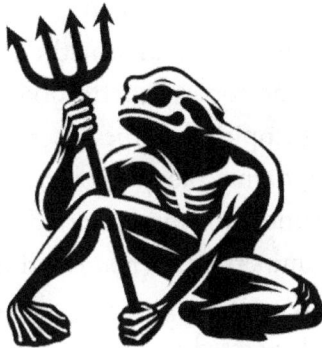

CHAPTER 4

Dr. Dave's Personal
Journeys

Psilocybin

Embarking on the journey within the mind's complex corridors demands a fortitude, liken to military training, martial arts, or extreme adventure sports. From this perspective, I sought to quell the tempest of existential disquiet that had plagued my psyche since childhood. The venture into the profound depths of psilocybin was not a decision made on a whim but a deliberate strategy to confront the inner tumult head-on.

My initiation into this realm started with the delicate practice of microdosing, a cautious exploration that honed the mind's acuity over the course of a year. Much like the meticulous calibration of a high-powered rifle, microdosing served as a method of fine-tuning perception, yielding a clarity and focus hitherto obscured by life's relentless barrages. Supported by empirical studies, such as the one published in the "Journal of Psychopharmacology" (Polito & Stevenson, 2019), this approach laid the groundwork for my mind to handle the potency of a total psychedelic immersion. When the time came to deepen my exploration, it was with a solemnity befitting a ritual. In the presence of a trusted comrade, I ingested a more substantial dose—3 grams of psilocybin mushrooms. This sacrament, consumed amongst the brilliance and beauty of the Michigan Upper Peninsula, was the key to unlocking the gate to profound self-confrontation.

As the psilocybin took effect, reality's rigidity dissolved, replaced by a vibrant energy that seemed to imbue every cell of my being. The natural world around me transformed into a tableau of otherworldly hues, the trees conducting a symphony of colors so intense they seemed to sing with an ethereal voice. Such synesthetic experiences are noted in transpersonal psychology as gateways to realms beyond ordinary consciousness (Grof, 1975), where one's sense of self is not just present but melded with the environment in a profound symbiosis.

This communion with nature culminated in a vision of a tree, its branches reaching out transforming into guiding arms, ushering me into a luminescent tunnel. It was a passage that transcended mere visual phenomena, a transcendentalist revelation in the vein of Emerson and Thoreau, where the sanctity of my intuition eclipsed the corporeal world's claims.

In this dimension, where linear time unraveled, I encountered entities that communicated through the universal language of emotion. Here, I was no longer Dave Ferruolo but a consciousness in communion with the ineffable. This fellowship of beings, encountered at the peak of my journey, imparted a sense of unity that transcended any camaraderie experienced in the human realm.

As the psilocybin's influence began to ebb, the departure from this communion was tinged with a sense of loss yet enriched by profound gratitude. Returning to the confines of my physical form, the experience left an indelible mark on my being.

The aftermath of the journey was not a cessation of life's challenges but rather a reframing of them. Laughter and smiles became more frequent visitors, spontaneous expressions of the joy the journey's echoes bestowed upon me. And yet, these experiences, as transformative as they were, underscored the indispensability of integration and professional guidance. The path traversed under the influence of psilocybin is not a one-time pilgrimage but an ongoing process of self-discovery and integration.

While the narrative of my psilocybin journey speaks to a profound and positive transformation, it is crucial to acknowledge that not all psychedelic experiences are unequivocally serene or enlightening. The realms of the psyche that such substances unveil can sometimes be tumultuous, confronting individuals with their deepest fears and insecurities. It's a stark reality that some voyages through the mind may surface as challenging, even harrowing experiences.

Yet, within these intense episodes, there is potential for significant growth. With the proper therapeutic support, these challenging experiences can become powerful catalysts for change, prompting deep psychological and emotional healing. The role of an experienced guide—a psychotherapist or counselor versed in psychedelic integration —becomes indispensable in these scenarios, transforming what might initially appear as a crisis into a pivotal moment of personal development. These complex dynamics highlight the necessity of approaching psychedelic therapy with caution, respect, and professional support to navigate and integrate the full spectrum of experiences that one might encounter.

Iboga

In the seclusion of a Mexican villa, the Pacific Ocean witnessed the ebbs and flows of its tides and the stirrings of the soul poised for the profound encounter with Ibogaine. Safety and spirituality coalesced in this sanctified haven, creating an environment ripe for the deep, introspective pursuit that awaited.

The ceremonial commencement of the Ibogaine experience was laced with a palpable reverence. This wasn't an endeavor taken lightly, underscored by the thorough medical vetting that prefaced the ingestion of the sacrament. Every detail of the space—from the reassuring solidity of IV stands to the softness of the mattresses—served as silent guardians for the journey ahead.

As the Ibogaine entered my system, reality began to undulate. Awaiting the onset of visions and hallucinations, I instead slipped into a profound introspective state. My companions may have traversed landscapes of vivid hallucinatory vistas, yet my passage was markedly different, echoing the diversity and personalized nature of psychedelic experiences.

Rather than external spectacles, I was drawn inward to a realm of existential revelation. This internal cinema was not a frivolous parade of memories but a demanding spiritual audit. As if the essence of Transcendentalism and the Platonic realm of forms were distilled into my very being, I engaged in a dialogue with my life's narrative. Like a series of vignettes, my subconscious presented scenes that demanded recognition before release, each acting as a stepping stone nearing an elusive transcendence.

This was not merely introspection but a reconstitution of self, embodying the Eastern philosophical principle of impermanence—each insight gained, and pattern shed was a conscious act of psychic evolution. As I emerged, the clarity gained was akin to a rebirth that transcended the mere conceptual understanding of my past self.

The experience was not merely a solitary journey but a shared rite of passage, with each of us submerged in the distinctive needs of our spiritual quest. Ibogaine, I realized, was a masterful teacher, leading me through the intricate chambers of the psyche with precise, tailored guidance and demanding respect and rigor in its approach.

This pilgrimage into the depths of the mind highlighted the inexorable flow of life's continuum, as depicted in Eastern traditions. The impermanence of our experience with Ibogaine laid the groundwork for a profound evolution, the ripples of which continue to resonate through the essence of our daily existence.

For those who might heed the call of Ibogaine, it's imperative to acknowledge the gravity of such an endeavor. It's a journey that necessitates physical readiness and psychological and spiritual fortitude. With this story, I impart a message that while the promise of transformation is genuine, it is only to be pursued with the scaffolding of professional guidance and a sanctuary that anchors the experience firmly in the realm of safety and sacredness.

5-MeO-DMT

In the mosaic of human experience, the profound encounter with 5-MeO-DMT, the "God Molecule," stands as a testament to the depths of consciousness—a venture not into the heart of darkness but into the cradle of light. The ceremonious introduction to this molecule commenced not with fanfare but with the solemnity befitting a sacrament. As the initial "handshake dose" permeated my being, it was as though I'd been invited to step across the threshold of a mystical portal, not dissimilar to the ancient shamanic traditions that sought communion with the divine.

The encounter with the ineffable commenced under the watchful eyes of guides whose presence was reassuring and vital. They were the seasoned navigators of these turbulent psychic seas, custodians of an experience that beckoned with the sublime allure of the numinous. In their hands, administering the subsequent doses became a rite of passage, each amplification of the substance drawing me deeper into the darkest corridors of my psyche—a maze where each twist and turn revealed new truths about my inner landscape.

With the progression of the experience, reality—once an intricate puzzle of tangible pieces— unraveled into something more fluid, a stream of consciousness that ebbed and flowed with the cosmic tides. The visions, neither terrifying nor ecstatic, carved their path through my awareness. They were the cartography of my subconscious, a revelation of the myriad paths that had brought me to this singular point in time and space. An inner voice beckoned that it was now time to go deeper.

As the second dose of 5-MeO-DMT entered my system, the room's meditative ambiance fell away, and I was thrust deeper into the uncharted waters of my consciousness. The initial tingling sensation escalated into a powerful vibratory force, enveloping me in a cocoon of sensory amplification. The geometric dance of black and white that had previously entertained my vision now morphed into a profound exploration of contrasts—light against dark, known against unknown, being against non-being.

This phase was akin to a tribulation of self-inquiry, each moment stretching into eternity, asking me to confront the shadows within. The feelings it evoked were intensely multifaceted: a confrontation with my deepest fears and a simultaneous recognition of my resilience. A coldness seemed to seep into every fiber of my being, a chilling reminder of the vastness in which I was suspended. It was not a physical coldness but an existential one, asking me to question the very nature of my being, the very nature of reality.

Emerging from the intensity of the second dose, the invitation for the third was a call to finality. I approached it with a mixture of trepidation and awe, aware that this was the threshold beyond which there would be no returning to the old self. The inhalation was a commitment, an acceptance of whatever lay beyond the veil.

The third dose marked the precipice of a profound departure—an explosive exodus from the familiar shores of self that I had navigated throughout my life. The reality I had known did not merely dissolve; it fractured violently, disintegrating into countless fragments of light and shadow. The disintegration was a visual spectacle and a visceral collapse of all that I had anchored myself to.

In this indescribable paradox, a visceral claustrophobia took hold—an acute, harrowing constriction, as if the entirety of the universe had conspired to compress upon my chest. The sensation was not metaphorical but brutally physical, an unbearable pressure that seemed to squeeze the very life from my lungs, riveting me to the core with a force that felt as though it could extinguish my fragile human existence. It was a psychological crucible, each breath a herculean task against the inexorable weight of creation bearing down upon me. The intensity was all-consuming, a suffocating grip that threatened to snuff out the vestiges of my consciousness.

At this moment, the terror was absolute, an all-encompassing fear that dwarfed any dread I had previously known. This was not the fear of the unknown but the terror of total annihilation—a confrontation with the stark possibility of non-existence. It bore down upon me with a merciless power beyond any force I could have conceived, as though cosmic forces were unraveling the very fabric of my being.

The only passage through this maelstrom of fear was surrender—a complete and utter capitulation to the experience. It demanded the abandonment of all attempts at control and the release of every shred of resistance. It was a submission in mind, spirit, and body, a letting go so profound that it felt akin to a small death, the ego dissolving in the face of the infinite. With every perceivable ounce of willpower, I submitted to turn the veracity of this terror into a curiosity and a willingness to explore. I relaxed into letting go, to accept whatever may come.

And then, in the heart of that storm, as I relinquished the grasping at control, the clinging to my perceived everything and my life, came the rapture. The release from the unbearable pressure.

It was instantaneous, a liberation so sudden and all-encompassing that it could only be described as ecstatic. The universe, which had seemed a relentless adversary, transformed into the ultimate liberator.

In that rapturous release, the dichotomy of light and darkness coalesced into a singular, boundless expanse. I was no longer confined by the physical limitations of the body; I became amorphous, expansive, a consciousness unbound by the temporal constraints of mortality. The surrender had not led to obliteration but had birthed an immersion into the totality of existence— a merging with the infinite, where the self was not lost but expanded into the vastness of the cosmos.

From this point, the journey was not a path back to where I had begun but a forward motion into a state of being that continues to ripple through the fibers of my life, leaving a permanent imprint of peace and unity that is woven into the very essence of who I am now. The terror and the subsequent rapture stand as profound testimonies to the transformative power of surrender in the face of the incomprehensible.

In this space, I was no longer a body, no longer a mere participant in the human experience. I became a point of consciousness, a singularity floating in the vastness of creation. I was in the presence of something far greater than myself, a force of such overwhelming love and peace that it transcended the need for form or substance.

This realm defied description, for it existed beyond the limitations of language and thought. It was a space where time curled upon itself, where the beginning and end of all things coalesced. I was at once the drop and the ocean, an individual soul reflecting the entire cosmos.

In the aftermath, as I returned to the room, to the here and now, the echoes of the journey remained. Laughter bubbled up from a place of pure joy, and tears streamed from a well of release I had not known was there. A profound clarity washed over me, bringing with it a peace that has since become a continuous undercurrent to my life.

The third dose was not simply a chapter in my life; it rewrote the entire book. Fear, negativity, and the burdens I had carried into the ceremony dissolved into a newfound purity of existence. The profound transformation was a rebirth, the emergence of a consciousness attuned to a deeper resonance, an attunement that has forever changed how I engage with the world.

This journey, through the stages of the second and third doses, was a voyage of discovery, an odyssey of the soul that stands as a beacon to the transformative power of 5-MeO-DMT when approached with reverence and courage. It is a tale not of escape but of return—a return to the essential unity of all things, a remembrance of the peace that dwells at the heart of existence.

The essence of the Bufo Toad (5-MeO-DMT) experience transcended the visual, touching something much more elemental. It was the Platonic ideal of experience, a confrontation with the fundamental nature of existence. In this journey of transformation, I found myself at once annihilated and reborn, a witness to the death of old paradigms and the birth of profound inner peace. It was the dance of Shiva, the destruction that precedes creation, the storm that yields to calm.

As I surfaced from the depths, the ineffable quality of this psychedelic voyage defied encapsulation. It was a narrative that strained against the confines of language, for how does one convey the true nature of a transformation so complete that it leaves the very bedrock of one's identity altered? In the aftermath, there was a lasting serenity, a continuous undercurrent of peace that permeated every facet of my existence. It was as if the mystical union with 5-MeO-DMT had gifted me an unshakable foundation, a peace that passed all understanding.

In reflection, the journey with 5-MeO-DMT was not an escape from reality but a deeper penetration into its very essence. It underscored the potential of psychedelics to catalyze profound personal growth when approached with the appropriate reverence, preparation, and guidance. The experience was not merely life-changing; it was life-affirming, offering a glimpse into the boundless potential of the human spirit to connect, transform, and transcend.

As the dust settles on this extraordinary voyage through consciousness, one finds themselves standing at the threshold of a new reality. The sacred space—the safe container where the journey unfolded—is now a cherished memory of the metamorphosis that occurred within. Yet, as the protective cocoon is left behind, the stark light of everyday life casts its relentless glare. The transition from the profound back to the profane is fraught with the complexity of reconciling who you were with who you have become.

This transformation echoes the metamorphosis of the caterpillar to the butterfly—a creature once bound to the earth, voraciously consuming nature, now reborn as an ethereal embodiment of grace and harmony. The chrysalis phase, a time of profound change, serves as a vivid metaphor for the psychic rebirth facilitated by 5-MeO-DMT. Yet, even after the emergence, the caterpillar's essence remains imprinted within the butterfly's cells.

Similarly, the neural pathways in our brain—those well-trodden roads and highways formed through a lifetime of habitual behavior—persist. Psychedelic experiences like 5-MeO-DMT have the power to expand these neural byways, offering glimpses of a transformed existence.

However, the deeply ingrained patterns of our former self are resilient; like ivy, they cling to the structures of our psyche, ready to ensnare us once more in the familiar embrace of who we were. Both Voltaire and Marcus Aurelius, through their writings, underscore the stoic philosophy of the necessity of diligent attention to our inner mental landscape, akin to a garden, where neglect can allow the weeds of negative thoughts to encroach upon and overwhelm the fruitful produce of a well-tended mind.

In my experience, the tension between the past, present, and future selves have proven to be a delicate dance. There lies a profound lesson in honoring the entirety of one's being—the person you were, who you are now, and who you are still becoming. It is a journey of acceptance, embracing every aspect of your transformation with compassion and without the burden of expectation.

Letting go of preconceived outcomes and severing future-based attachments became an act of liberation. The key is to reside in a state of being that is fluid and open to the unfolding quintessence of life. It is an ongoing process of integration, a nurturing of the emergent self, allowing for the continuous evolution of the psyche.

The journey does not conclude with the psychedelic experience itself; it is merely the beginning. As one navigates the complexities of life post-transformation, it is imperative to take the necessary time for integration. This means mindfully acknowledging the resurgence of old patterns, tenderly steering them to the new paths uncovered by the psychedelic experience.

To evolve is to embrace change in its entirety, allowing the self to unfurl at its own pace. It is a gentle unfolding, a bloom that cannot be rushed. In honoring the entirety of this process, we not only accept the transformation but learn to thrive within it, carrying forward the gifts of our journeys into the intricate dance of life.

CHAPTER 5

What Are Psychedelics?

In the recesses of human history, there exists a category of substances that have held humanity in thrall—a group of compounds that have, for eons, beckoned to the depths of our psyche and awakened the slumbering essence of our consciousness. These are the psychedelics, a term coined not merely to describe a class of chemicals but to encapsulate the very essence of a transcendent journey into the uncharted realms of the human experience. In this chapter, we embark on a quest that transcends the ordinary delving into the enigmatic world of these compounds, often labeled as hallucinogens. They are more than mere substances; they are the alchemical keys to the extraordinary unfurling within our minds.

At the heart of this exploration lies a paradox—psychedelics, the so-called "hallucinogens," possess a remarkable gift. They are the alchemists of the psyche, capable of transporting us beyond the confines of our mundane senses, unlocking doors to vistas of consciousness that defy the rational, the linear, and the ordinary. They invite us to gaze into the abyss of our own being, where perception, cognition, and emotion fuse into a kaleidoscope of experience, where the boundaries of self-dissolve like morning mist under the rising sun.

In the ancient wisdom of etymology, the word "psychedelic" emerges as a compound of "psyche," signifying the soul or mind, and "deloun," meaning to reveal or manifest. It is a term that carries a profound implication—the notion that these substances have the power not only to reveal the hidden recesses of our psyche but also to unveil the very essence of our being. They are not mere chemicals; they are the catalysts of profound revelation, the keys that open the gates to the extraordinary depths of our minds.

This chapter beckons you to embark on a journey of profundity, where words alone cannot suffice to convey the magnitude of what lies ahead. It transcends the mundane and invites you to peer beyond the ordinary veils of perception, to question the very fabric of reality, and to dance at the precipice of existence itself.

As we delve deeper into this exploration, we must remember that psychedelics are not merely substances; they are the alchemical elixirs of transformation, the sacred sacraments of indigenous wisdom, and the catalysts for profound revelations that have shaped cultures, ignited revolutions, and transformed lives. In the chapters that follow, we shall not only unveil the historical roots of these substances but also illuminate their contemporary resurgence—a resurgence not only in the laboratories of science but in the very heart of human consciousness.

An Array of Compounds

Within the vastness of psychedelics, a captivating spectrum of compounds awaits exploration, each wielding its unique signature upon the human psyche. As we embark on this comprehensive journey through the realm of psychedelic substances, it is essential to delve into their individual nuances and applications, particularly concerning combat-related psychological and emotional issues. This thorough examination will not only elucidate the potential of these substances but also underscore their relevance in the context of healing for combat veterans.

Ketamine, initially designed as an anesthetic agent, has emerged as a promising and innovative therapeutic tool for combat veterans contending with the burdens of trauma-related disorders. Recent research illuminates the potential of low-dose ketamine infusion therapy to deliver swift and tangible relief from symptoms of depression, anxiety, and post-traumatic stress disorder (PTSD). What sets ketamine apart from classic psychedelics is not only its distinct pharmacological profile but also its capacity to induce a state of dissociation, a key element in its therapeutic prowess. This chapter seeks to comprehensively explore the multifaceted nature of ketamine therapy, shedding light on its unique mechanism of action, clinical applications, and its profound impact on veterans' mental health.

Ketamine's mechanism of action distinguishes it from the classic psychedelics we've discussed earlier. Instead of targeting serotonin receptors, as seen in substances like psilocybin and LSD, ketamine operates through the modulation of glutamate receptors, specifically the N-methyl-D-aspartate (NMDA) receptors. This action results in a cascade of effects that trigger neuroplasticity, synaptic remodeling, and a rapid shift in the brain's functional connectivity.

One of ketamine's unique attributes is its ability to induce dissociation, a state where the individual becomes detached from their usual sense of self and surroundings. While this phenomenon might sound unsettling, within the context of therapeutic ketamine sessions, it is a crucial element for healing. By dissociating, patients are afforded a degree of emotional distance from their traumatic memories, allowing them to revisit and process these experiences in a controlled and safe therapeutic setting. This process can lead to emotional breakthroughs, increased insight, and a gradual desensitization to trauma-related triggers.

Research has consistently shown that ketamine infusion therapy can produce rapid and substantial relief from symptoms of depression, anxiety, and PTSD. Unlike traditional antidepressant medications that may take weeks or even months to take effect, ketamine often provides relief within hours or days of administration. For combat veterans who may be grappling with immediate and intense distress, this rapid response can be life-changing.

It's crucial to emphasize that ketamine therapy should only be administered under the supervision of trained healthcare professionals in a clinical setting. The dosing, timing, and patient monitoring are carefully managed to ensure both safety and efficacy. The importance of a supportive therapeutic environment cannot be overstated, as it allows veterans to navigate the intense and sometimes challenging emotional terrain that ketamine therapy can unveil.

Ketamine has emerged as a powerful and novel therapeutic tool in the arsenal of treatments available for combat veterans struggling with trauma-related disorders. Its unique mechanism of action, capacity to induce dissociation, and rapid relief of symptoms make it a valuable option for those in need of immediate relief and emotional healing. However, it is essential that ketamine therapy is administered by qualified professionals who can guide veterans through this transformative process, offering them a pathway to healing and resilience on their post-combat journey.

MDMA, known colloquially as ecstasy or Molly, has increasingly captured the spotlight within the realm of psychotherapy, offering new hope for individuals, particularly combat veterans, grappling with the harrowing effects of post-traumatic stress disorder (PTSD). This chapter delves into the multifaceted nature of MDMA-assisted therapy, shedding light on its mechanism of action, clinical applications, and the transformative potential it holds for those seeking to navigate the turbulent waters of trauma-related issues.

MDMA's unique mechanism of action sets it apart from traditional psychedelics. Unlike substances such as psilocybin or LSD, which primarily target serotonin receptors, MDMA primarily affects the release and reuptake of neurotransmitters, including serotonin, norepinephrine, and dopamine. This distinctive pharmacological profile results in an altered state of consciousness characterized by heightened emotional openness, increased empathy, and reduced fear and defensiveness.

The empathogenic quality of MDMA is at the core of its therapeutic potential. When administered within the structured and supportive environment of psychotherapy sessions, MDMA fosters a profound sense of emotional connection and trust between the patient and therapist. This empathogenic state allows combat veterans to traverse the often treacherous terrain of their traumatic experiences with greater ease and resilience.

MDMA-assisted therapy provides combat veterans with a unique opportunity to confront and process their trauma-related issues. The drug's empathogenic effects create a safe space for individuals to delve deep into their emotional landscapes, allowing them to communicate openly about their experiences, fears, and insecurities. This uninhibited communication promotes a therapeutic alliance built on trust and understanding, which is foundational for effective trauma processing.

The promise of MDMA in psychotherapy is not merely speculative; it is supported by a growing body of evidence. Rigorous clinical trials have consistently demonstrated its efficacy in reducing PTSD symptoms. Notably, the Food and Drug Administration (FDA) has recognized the potential of MDMA-assisted therapy, granting it breakthrough therapy designation for the treatment of PTSD. This designation underscores the urgency and importance of further research into this innovative approach to healing.

MDMA-assisted therapy represents a transformative path forward for combat veterans and individuals who have PTSD. Its empathogenic qualities, ability to foster open communication, and promising results in clinical trials have positioned it as a groundbreaking tool in the field of psychotherapy. As research continues to unfold, MDMA has the potential to offer hope, healing, and a renewed sense of well-being to those who have endured the profound effects of trauma.

Please note that this information is provided for educational purposes, and individuals seeking MDMA-assisted therapy should do so under the guidance of trained professionals in a legal and clinical context.

Ibogaine, derived from the African Tabernanthe iboga plant, Ibogaine is a substance that has garnered attention for its unique and intense psychedelic properties. Although its study is not as extensive as some other psychedelics, it holds promise in addressing substance use disorders—a challenge frequently intertwined with combat-related mental health issues. In this chapter, we delve into the complex and multifaceted nature of Ibogaine, exploring its potential as a therapeutic tool, its mechanisms of action, and its relevance for combat veterans' recovery and integration.

Ibogaine's origins trace back to the Bwiti religious tradition in Central Africa, where it has been used for centuries in spiritual and healing rituals. This deep-rooted cultural context underscores the substance's profound role in altering consciousness and facilitating introspection.

One of the defining characteristics of Ibogaine is the intensity of the psychedelic experience it induces. Unlike some other psychedelics, Ibogaine is known for its extended duration, often spanning many hours. Users report vivid visions, deep introspection, and a sense of being confronted with their innermost thoughts and emotions. This intensity can be both challenging and transformative, making Ibogaine a substance that demands careful consideration and supervision.

Ibogaine's potential as a tool to address substance use disorders, including addiction to opioids and other substances, has been a subject of growing interest. Research suggests that Ibogaine may have a unique ability to disrupt addiction patterns by resetting neural pathways and facilitating a deep psychological reckoning with the roots of addiction. While this is a promising avenue, it's essential to acknowledge that ibogaine treatment is not without risks and should only be administered by experienced professionals in a controlled and medically supervised environment.

For combat veterans struggling with substance misuse as a coping mechanism for the traumas they've endured, Ibogaine offers a glimpse of hope. Its potential to address addiction at its core, coupled with its capacity for profound introspection, aligns with the complex needs of individuals who have experienced the rigors of combat. However, it's imperative to underscore the importance of safety and professional guidance when considering ibogaine therapy.

While Ibogaine shows promise, it is crucial to recognize that its therapeutic potential is still being explored. Rigorous research and clinical trials are necessary to better understand its efficacy, safety, and long-term effects. As we navigate the evolving landscape of psychedelic therapy for combat veterans, Ibogaine remains an enigmatic yet potentially transformative ally in the battle against substance use disorders and the healing journey toward mental well-being.

Psilocybin, the active compound residing within the mystical confines of magic mushrooms, beckons us to embark on a journey into the enigmatic realms of altered consciousness. With a rich historical background woven through various cultural and spiritual traditions, psilocybin emerges as a potential beacon of hope for combat veterans grappling with the weight of combat-related psychological and emotional burdens, particularly post-traumatic stress disorder (PTSD) and depression. This chapter undertakes a comprehensive exploration of the multifaceted dimensions of psilocybin-assisted therapy, encompassing its historical significance, mechanisms of action, clinical applications, and the compelling results emanating from recent clinical trials.

The historical and cultural significance of psilocybin-containing mushrooms spans millennia, encapsulating a profound journey through human civilizations. Indigenous cultures around the world have held these mushrooms in awe and reverence, weaving them into the fabric of their spiritual and healing traditions. This chapter unfolds the historical depth of this relationship, revealing the enduring legacy of psilocybin across time and place.

One of the most iconic examples of the historical use of psilocybin can be found in the indigenous cultures of Mesoamerica, particularly the Aztecs and the Maya. In the Codex Madrid, an Aztec manuscript dating back to the 16th century, depictions of mushrooms closely resembling Psilocybe mexicana, a psilocybin-containing species, are evident. These sacred mushrooms were believed to be a means of communing with the gods and gaining spiritual insights. Similarly, the Maya civilization revered "teonanácatl," or "God's flesh," as they called the mushrooms. They believed that partaking in these sacraments connected them to the divine and facilitated prophetic visions.

Beyond Mesoamerica, psilocybin-containing mushrooms have played integral roles in the spiritual practices of various indigenous cultures worldwide. The Mazatec people of Mexico have long used Psilocybe cubensis, commonly known as "sacred mushrooms," in their healing rituals and shamanic traditions. In the Amazon rainforest, indigenous tribes like the Shipibo-Conibo and the Santo Daime have incorporated psilocybin-containing fungi into their ayahuasca ceremonies, believing that these mushrooms aid in the exploration of spiritual realms and the healing of the mind and soul.

The modern world witnessed a resurgence of interest in psilocybin during the mid-20th century when Western researchers and counter-culture figures encountered these mushrooms. Notable figures like Terence McKenna and Timothy Leary became advocates for their use, touting their potential to expand consciousness and explore the depths of the human mind. This revival sparked further research into psilocybin's therapeutic potential, leading to contemporary clinical trials and its recognition as a powerful tool for psychological healing.

The historical and cultural reverence for psilocybin has persisted through time and continues to evolve. In the present day, a renaissance of psilocybin research is unfolding, with rigorous scientific studies exploring its therapeutic applications. Psilocybin-assisted therapy is becoming a beacon of hope for individuals suffering from mental health issues, including combat veterans grappling with the traumas of war.

In the realm of mental health care, psilocybin has emerged as a transformative tool for combat veterans grappling with the profound wounds of war—PTSD and depression. This chapter explores psilocybin's journey to becoming a beacon of hope for veterans contending with complex combat-related psychological and emotional challenges.

Combat veterans are often resistant to conventional treatments. This demands innovative healing approaches. Psilocybin-assisted therapy marks a seismic shift in mental health care. Psilocybin offers a transformative path beyond traditional interventions. Guided by skilled therapists in a secure setting, veterans embark on introspective journeys.

Psilocybin-assisted therapy is not simply a journey of the mind; it is a profound and intentional process that operates through a specific mechanism of action, ultimately leading to therapeutic change. In this section, we will delve into the intriguing process by which psilocybin induces transformative experiences and facilitates healing for combat veterans.

The Dance of Serotonin Receptors: At the core of psilocybin's mechanism of action lies its interaction with serotonin receptors in the brain. Psilocybin is converted into psilocin upon ingestion, and it is psilocin that primarily engages with the brain's serotonin receptors, particularly the 5-HT2A receptor. This interaction sets in motion a cascade of events that culminate in the psychedelic experience.

Breaking Down Default Mode Network (DMN): One of the key effects of psilocybin is the suppression of the default mode network (DMN) in the brain. The DMN is responsible for our sense of self, autobiographical thinking, and the incessant mental chatter that often characterizes our waking state. Psilocybin disrupts this network, leading to a state of ego dissolution, where individuals temporarily lose their sense of self and experience a feeling of interconnectedness with the world.

Enhancing Neuroplasticity and Connectivity: As the DMN relaxes its grip, the brain's connectivity patterns shift. Psilocybin encourages previously separated brain regions to communicate more freely, leading to increased neuroplasticity and the formation of new neural connections. This heightened connectivity may underlie the increased introspection and novel insights experienced during therapy sessions.

Confronting Trauma and Emotional Processing: With the ego temporarily set aside, individuals undergoing psilocybin therapy can confront their traumatic memories and emotions in a more direct and unfiltered manner. This emotional processing is a central component of the therapeutic journey. Veterans can re-experience their traumas in a safe and supportive environment, enabling them to process and reframe these memories, often leading to profound healing.

Trained therapists play a pivotal role in guiding veterans through the psilocybin experience. Their expertise helps individuals navigate the sometimes intense and emotionally charged terrain of the psychedelic journey. The therapist's presence offers reassurance and support, facilitating the therapeutic process.

The insights gained during psilocybin sessions are not confined to the therapy room. Veterans work with their therapists to integrate these newfound perspectives and emotional breakthroughs into their daily lives. This ongoing process ensures that the healing experienced during therapy extends beyond the sessions themselves.

Psilocybin-assisted therapy employs a unique mechanism of action that disrupts the default mode network, enhances brain connectivity, and promotes emotional processing. Trained therapists provide essential support in guiding veterans through this transformative journey, ultimately leading to therapeutic change that extends into their post-combat lives. Psilocybin offers a comprehensive approach to healing, addressing the complex and deeply rooted wounds of war with newfound hope and resilience.

LSD, originating from the synthesis of ergot fungi, has a storied past as a catalyst for revolutions in thought and art. When harnessed within therapeutic contexts, it has the potential to facilitate deep introspection and emotional release, offering new avenues for healing and personal growth, including its implications for combat veterans. In this section, we will delve into LSD's mechanism of action, its evolving landscape in therapy, and its potential to benefit those who have served in the military.

LSD's profound effects stem from its interaction with serotonin receptors in the brain, particularly the 5-HT2A receptor. This interaction alters the usual patterns of serotonin transmission, leading to profound alterations in perception, cognition, and emotional experience. These shifts in brain activity are thought to underlie the therapeutic potential of LSD.

Within the therapeutic setting, LSD can be a potent catalyst for introspection. Veterans who have experienced the horrors of war often carry emotional burdens that resist conventional therapeutic approaches. LSD can help them access and confront these deeply buried emotions and memories, offering a unique pathway to healing.

While rigorous research on LSD's application for combat veterans is ongoing, anecdotal evidence suggests its potential. Veterans have reported profound personal insights, emotional release, and a sense of catharsis during LSD-assisted therapy. These experiences have the potential to foster personal growth, resilience, and a newfound perspective on their traumatic experiences.

Research into LSD's efficacy in treating combat-related mental health issues is still in its infancy. Preliminary studies and ongoing clinical trials are exploring its potential benefits, but more comprehensive research is needed to establish its place within the therapeutic toolkit for veterans.

The legal status of LSD varies widely across different jurisdictions. In some places, it is strictly controlled or prohibited, while in others, it may be used in clinical research or under specific circumstances. Combat veterans and therapists must be aware of the legal landscape in their respective regions when considering LSD-assisted therapy.

LSD has a rich history as a catalyst for profound shifts in consciousness and thought. Within the realm of therapy, it holds promise for combat veterans struggling with the burdens of trauma. While the anecdotal evidence suggests its potential for healing and personal growth, ongoing research is necessary to fully understand its efficacy and establish its place within the therapeutic toolkit. Additionally, the legal status of LSD must be carefully considered in any therapeutic context involving this substance.

DMT and 5-MeO-DMT. In the context of psychotherapeutic potential, particularly for combat veterans contending with PTSD, moral injury, and substance use, the exploration of both DMT and 5-MeO-DMT holds profound relevance. While DMT is often associated with intricate, vivid visions and intense emotional experiences, 5-MeO-DMT, primarily sourced from the secretion of the Bufo Alvarius toad, is heralded for its more ineffable and overwhelming sense of oneness or nonduality.

Both DMT and 5-MeO-DMT fall under the category of tryptamine psychedelics and share molecular similarities with serotonin, thereby exerting significant effects on serotonin receptors throughout the brain. However, their phenomenological impacts diverge substantially, a variance that may also reflect differing receptor bindings and neural activation patterns.

5-MeO-DMT's mechanism is not merely an amplification of DMT's effects but represents a distinct experiential profile. It is believed that 5-MeO-DMT has a higher affinity for the 5-HT1A receptor, which could play a role in its unique ability to induce profound ego-dissolving experiences, a phenomenon often termed "ego death." This can result in the sensation of merging with the universe or the obliteration of normal perceptual boundaries, giving rise to a mystical experience of oneness that is described as being beyond words.

The notion of ego death entails the temporary dismantlement of the ego— the individual's sense of self and identity. In therapeutic settings, this disruption is hypothesized to enable combat veterans to observe their traumas, fears, and emotional pains without the typical defensive structures that the ego upholds. This can create a space for profound psychological shifts, potentially allowing for the reconsolidation of traumatic memories and the fostering of a new perspective on life and identity.

The rebirth that follows is often described by veterans as a sense of awakening—like emerging from a cocoon with a fresh perspective that transcends previous limiting beliefs and traumas. This awakening is not simply a return to baseline but is characterized by a newfound sense of connectivity with oneself, others, and the world at large.

5-MeO-DMT's potential to catalyze a rapid and profound awakening, with enduring effects from a single session, aligns with the urgent need for effective therapeutic interventions in combat veterans who often endure chronic and treatment-resistant conditions. By transiently inducing a state in which normal cognitive processing is suspended, 5-MeO-DMT may facilitate a therapeutic window wherein individuals can confront deep-seated issues without their customary psychological defenses.

For the transformation to be lasting, the experiences with 5-MeO-DMT must be integrated into the individual's life. This process is essential, especially for veterans who might have faced their deepest vulnerabilities during the experience. Integration involves making sense of the experience, attributing meaning to it, and applying insights gained to one's life. The role of trained facilitators is critical in this phase, guiding veterans through this delicate period of psychic reorganization.

The therapeutic promise of DMT and, notably, 5-MeO-DMT in psychedelic-assisted psychotherapy is profound, resonating deeply with the psychological and spiritual exigencies of combat veterans. My own encounters with these substances can attest to their formidable potency. The rapid immersion into an intense existential state, akin to the universe itself collapsing upon my chest, demands skilled navigation and a comprehensive therapeutic framework that acknowledges the profound sacrifices and experiences of veterans.

These experiences, including my own grappling with a near-overwhelming claustrophobia followed by an eventual surrender to the rapture of rebirth, underscore the necessity of a multifaceted approach. This approach not only honors the journey of the individual but also facilitates a transformative realignment with their sense of self and place in the cosmos, paving the way for healing and self-discovery.

The empirical grounding of these substances is still under construction in the scientific community, but each narrative of transformation and healing adds a vital piece to the puzzle. As research evolves and clinical protocols are refined, DMT and 5-MeO-DMT stand as potential keys to unlocking new pathways to healing for those who have served in combat and now seek peace on the home front.

Entheogens: The exploration of entheogens like Ayahuasca and mescaline takes us into the heart of indigenous traditions, where these substances are not merely chemical compounds, but sacred brews believed to open doorways to spiritual dimensions. For combat veterans who often return with wounds that are more than physical—traumas that are both psychological and, in many cases, spiritual—these traditional medicines offer a tantalizing glimpse of potential healing.

Ayahuasca is a mixture of the Banisteriopsis caapi vine and other plants that typically contain the powerful psychoactive compound DMT. Its use in Amazonian shamanic practices is deeply ritualized, intended for spiritual awakening and healing. Ayahuasca sessions often lead to intense introspection, offering veterans a space to confront and reconcile inner turmoil. The visions and emotional release that accompany an Ayahuasca journey can be integral in the process of addressing PTSD and moral injury, often unearthing subconscious narratives that need to be processed.

Mescaline is found in the peyote cactus and in San Pedro and Peruvian torch cacti; mescaline has been used for thousands of years by Native American communities for spiritual purposes. Mescaline's effects can range from deep euphoria to profound life-altering insights, which aid veterans in recontextualizing their experiences and integrating them into a broader understanding of self and the world.

Both Ayahuasca and mescaline invite an individual to step into a space where the sacred and the self-intersect. The profound spiritual experiences induced by these entheogens can lead to a sense of interconnectedness with all things, a perspective that is often occluded by the traumas of war. It's important to note that these substances are not without their risks and should not be approached casually. The guidance of experienced facilitators, often shamanic practitioners in traditional contexts, is crucial for navigating the potential challenges and revelations these experiences may bring.

The research on Ayahuasca and mescaline within the context of combat veterans is still emergent, yet anecdotal evidence suggests a potential for these substances to act as catalysts for emotional and psychological healing. In therapeutic settings, the integration of the profound experiences facilitated by these entheogens is as important as the experiences themselves. It is through careful integration that veterans can begin to reconstruct their sense of self and purpose, often finding a newfound peace that allows them to move forward in life with greater resilience and understanding.

Cultural and spiritual traditions across the globe have long recognized the capacity of psychedelics to unlock dimensions of the mind that typically lie beyond the reach of everyday awareness. The use of such substances can be traced back to ancient practices, which were often entwined with the quest for wisdom and the expansion of consciousness.

For example, within the shamanistic practices of indigenous tribes, plants such as Ayahuasca and peyote are considered sacred, with their ingestion being a conduit for healing and for receiving guidance from the spirit world. These experiences are not viewed merely as the effects of psychoactive substances but as spiritual journeys, providing insight and resolution to personal and communal issues.

The Eleusinian Mysteries of Greece have their own historical entwinement of psychedelics with spiritual questing. Here, the initiates would consume a potion known as 'kykeon,' which is thought to have contained psychoactive agents. This ritual was integral to experiencing the cycle of death and rebirth, a symbolic journey into the underworld that granted profound philosophical insights.

In the modern context, psychedelics are being revisited not only for their therapeutic potential but also for their ability to engender a profound connection with something greater than oneself, often described as a sense of oneness with the universe. This facet of the psychedelic experience resonates with many spiritual traditions, which speak of the dissolution of ego and the attainment of enlightenment.

Understanding these substances within their historical and cultural contexts enriches the therapeutic process. It underscores the point that healing is a medical endeavor and a multifaceted journey that can encompass spiritual growth and existential understanding.

Psychedelics have thus emerged as potent facilitators in this process, revealing new perspectives and dimensions of the human psyche. As we delve deeper into their storied past, we find an array of effects on the brain and a mirror reflecting the perennial human pursuit of knowledge, wholeness, and the sacred. This framing may not only illuminate the path for those seeking healing but also inspire a deeper appreciation for the profound wisdom encoded in cultural and spiritual practices of yore.

Contemplating these journeys, one might be encouraged to approach psychedelics with a sense of reverence and openness to the transformative experiences they can provide. It is essential to acknowledge their power and to navigate their use with care, ideally within the context of guided therapy and with respect for the historical wisdom that informs contemporary practice.

CHAPTER 6

Historical Use and Recent Resurgence

In this chapter, we delve into the rich history of psychedelic substances and their recent resurgence, with a particular focus on their relevance to combat veterans and their families. Our exploration will span historical perspectives, psychological insights, philosophical contemplations, and spiritual dimensions, providing a comprehensive overview of the fascinating journey of psychedelics.

Historical Perspectives

Indigenous cultures worldwide have a rich and enduring history of utilizing psychedelic substances within their spiritual and healing practices. This section investigates the profound significance of these practices and their connection to psychedelic substances.

Native American Peyote Rituals: Among Indigenous cultures in North America, particularly among the Native American Church, the peyote cactus (Lophophora williamsii) holds a sacred place in religious ceremonies. The use of peyote as a sacrament allows participants to embark on journeys of profound spiritual significance. It is believed that the consumption of peyote facilitates communion with the divine, connects individuals to their ancestors, and offers insights into the mysteries of existence.

Amazonian Ayahuasca Traditions: Across the Amazon rainforests, Ayahuasca ceremonies have been a cornerstone of Indigenous traditions for centuries. Ayahuasca, a potent psychedelic brew prepared from the Banisteriopsis caapi vine and the Psychotria viridis plant, plays a central role in these ceremonies. Shamans, or Ayahuasqueros, lead participants in consuming Ayahuasca, guiding them through intense and transformative experiences. The purpose is to communicate with ancestral spirits, diagnose illnesses, and gain deep insights into the human psyche (Jay, 2019).

Beyond Indigenous cultures, shamanic traditions worldwide have integrated psychedelics into their rituals for generations. This section sheds light on the role of shamans as spiritual guides and healers who utilize psychedelics for their profound effects.

Shamans and Altered States: Shamans, regarded as intermediaries between the spiritual and earthly realms, employ psychedelic substances like psilocybin-containing mushrooms and Ayahuasca to induce altered states of consciousness. These altered states are believed to facilitate communication with spirits, enabling shamans to provide guidance, healing, and insights to their communities. These practices are deeply rooted in the belief that the spiritual and physical worlds are interconnected.

Ancient civilizations also recognized the transformative potential of psychedelic substances. In the heart of ancient Greece, the Eleusinian Mysteries stood as one of the most revered and enigmatic religious traditions. At its core was a profound and mysterious potion known as the *Kykeon.* The Eleusinian Mysteries used Kykeon for the transformative experiences it bestowed upon its participants.

The Eleusinian Mysteries were a series of initiation ceremonies and rituals held annually in the city of Eleusis, near Athens. These sacred rites, dedicated to the goddesses Demeter and Persephone, attracted thousands of participants from all walks of life, from commoners to philosophers.

At the heart of these ceremonies was the Kykeon, a brew shrouded in secrecy and mystique. The exact composition of Kykeon remains a subject of debate among scholars, but it is believed to have contained barley, water, and perhaps other botanical ingredients. What set Kykeon apart was not its ingredients but its transformative effects.

Those who partook in the Eleusinian Mysteries and consumed the Kykeon reported profound and mystical experiences. Participants described encounters with divine entities, a heightened sense of spiritual awareness, and a deep connection to the mysteries of existence (Hoffman et al., 2008). It was as though the boundaries between the earthly and the divine had dissolved, allowing individuals to transcend their ordinary perceptions of reality.

The Eleusinian Mysteries were not exclusive to a particular class or group; they welcomed participants from diverse backgrounds. Philosophers like Plato and Aristotle were said to have undergone initiation into the Mysteries, attesting to the universal appeal of the experiences facilitated by the Kykeon.

The cultural and spiritual impact of the Eleusinian Mysteries was profound. They influenced art, literature, and philosophy in ancient Greece, leaving an indelible mark on the collective consciousness of the time. Even today, the exact nature of the experiences induced by the Kykeon remains a subject of fascination and inquiry.

The Eleusinian Mysteries and their use of the Kykeon offer a glimpse into the spiritual and mystical dimensions of psychedelic substances in ancient Greece. The transformative experiences reported by those who participated in these sacred rituals underscore the enduring human quest for transcendence, spiritual awakening, and a deeper understanding of the mysteries of existence.

Vedic Rituals and the Plant "Soma": In ancient Indian spirituality and Vedic rituals, the sacred plant known as "Soma" occupies a place of profound significance. This section delves into the mystical realm of Soma, exploring its pivotal role in the spiritual practices of ancient India and the enduring impact it had on the evolution of Hinduism.

At the heart of this narrative is the Rigveda, one of the oldest and most revered texts in Hinduism. Within its verses, there are numerous references to Soma, a plant believed to possess divine properties. These references shed light on the central role of Soma in Vedic rituals and spiritual experiences.

Soma was not merely a botanical specimen; it was revered as a sacred and divine elixir, often described as the "nectar of the gods." The preparation of Soma likely involved the extraction of its psychoactive properties, which were believed to enable direct communion with the divine realm. Soma was considered a bridge between the earthly and the celestial, a substance that facilitated communication with the gods themselves.

The consumption of Soma was not a casual act but a profoundly spiritual one. Partaking in Soma rituals was thought to induce altered states of consciousness, leading to transcendent experiences. Practitioners believed that through Soma, they could transcend the limitations of the physical world and attain direct knowledge of the divine mysteries.

Soma's importance extends beyond its psychoactive effects. It symbolized the very essence of divinity and was central to the spiritual life of ancient Indian practitioners. The act of preparing, offering, and consuming Soma was a sacred and transformative ritual, embodying the deep connection between humans and the divine.

The legacy of Soma rituals reverberates through the annals of Hinduism. While the exact identity of the plant referred to as Soma remains a subject of scholarly debate, its spiritual significance is unquestionable. Soma rituals and the profound experiences associated with them played a pivotal role in shaping the religious and philosophical landscape of ancient India, leaving an enduring imprint on the beliefs and practices of Hinduism.

The references to Soma in the Rigveda offer a window into the spiritual and mystical dimensions of Vedic rituals in ancient India. Soma's status as a divine elixir, capable of facilitating transcendent experiences and direct communion with the divine, underscores the profound and timeless human quest for spiritual awakening and a deeper connection with the sacred.

Changing Tides

The mid-20th century stands as a pivotal juncture in the evolving narrative of psychedelics. It was a turning point marked by notable researchers, societal concerns, and regulatory shifts, ultimately leading to the suppression and stigmatization of these substances.

During the mid-20th century, a profound shift occurred in the realm of psychedelic research. Notable figures such as Albert Hofmann, Aldous Huxley and Timothy Leary embarked on a journey of exploration, peering into the untapped therapeutic potential of these enigmatic substances. These studies, concentrating on LSD, began to unveil the transformative therapeutic benefits of psychedelics, offering hope for those grappling with psychological and psychiatric conditions.

Among the most compelling discoveries was the ability of psychedelics to address a spectrum of psychological and psychiatric conditions. These substances exhibited a remarkable capacity to alleviate the burden of depression, providing individuals with a profound sense of relief from the weight of their emotional struggles. Anxiety, often an unwelcome companion in the lives of many, was also shown to yield to the therapeutic embrace of psychedelics, as individuals experienced a profound sense of calm and a reduction in anxiety symptoms.

In the realm of substance use disorders, psychedelics held promise as tools for breaking the cycle of addiction. It was observed that individuals grappling with various forms of substance dependency, whether on alcohol, tobacco, or other substances, experienced a shift in their relationship with addiction. Psychedelics facilitated a deep, introspective journey, allowing individuals to confront the underlying causes of their addictive behaviors and providing them with an opportunity for profound transformation.

The therapeutic benefits observed in these studies heralded a paradigm shift in the understanding of psychedelics. They were no longer solely perceived as countercultural agents or tools of exploration but emerged as potential allies in the field of mental health treatment. The profound impact of these substances on psychological and psychiatric conditions signaled a new frontier in therapy, where the mind could be guided through healing and self-discovery by the therapeutic embrace of psychedelics.

This era of research offered a glimpse into the transformative potential of psychedelics, setting the stage for further exploration and the recent resurgence of interest in these substances as therapeutic tools.

However, the growing interest in psychedelics also gave rise to societal concerns. Some individuals began using these substances recreationally, leading to concerns about misuse, adverse effects, and the potential for harm.

The scheduling and subsequent classification of psychedelics as Schedule I substances under the Controlled Substances Act of 1970 in the United States represented a significant shift in the legal and regulatory landscape. Several key players and underlying motives contributed to this pivotal decision, which had profound consequences for the perception and use of these substances.

As interest in psychedelics grew during the mid-20th century, so did concerns about their misuse. Individuals began using these substances recreationally, often in uncontrolled settings and without proper guidance. This raised alarm bells among both the public and policymakers, who feared the potential for misuse and the associated adverse effects.

The era was marked by a broader cultural shift, with concerns about moral values and social norms coming to the forefront. Psychedelics were sometimes associated with counterculture movements that challenged conventional values, and this association contributed to a negative perception of these substances. Some religious groups that used psychedelics in their rituals also faced scrutiny and legal challenges.

Political pressure to demonstrate a tough stance on drugs influenced the decision to regulate psychedelics more strictly. The so-called "war on drugs" was gaining momentum during this period, and taking a strong stance against all drug use, including psychedelics, became a political priority.

Concerns about the potential harm associated with the use of psychedelics were a driving force behind the regulatory changes. Reports of adverse reactions and "bad trips" garnered attention, fueling fears about the unpredictable nature of psychedelic experiences.

Limited scientific understanding of psychedelics at the time contributed to the decision to schedule these substances. The complexity of psychedelic experiences, as well as their potential benefits and risks, was not well-researched or well-understood. This lack of knowledge made it difficult to assess the true impact and potential therapeutic value of these substances.

In response to these concerns and pressures, regulatory changes were enacted to tighten control over psychedelics. The Controlled Substances Act of 1970 placed many psychedelics, including LSD and psilocybin, in the most restrictive legal category, Schedule I. This classification effectively made them illegal for most purposes, including medical research and therapeutic use.

The decision to schedule psychedelics as Schedule I substances was influenced by a complex interplay of social, political, and public health factors. It represented a turning point in the legal and societal treatment of these substances, setting the stage for decades of restricted access and limited research opportunities.

The classification of psychedelics as Schedule I substances had profound implications. It not only restricted their use in research but also contributed to their suppression and stigmatization in society at large. Psychedelics, once seen as promising tools for therapy and exploration of the mind, became associated with counterculture movements and a perceived threat to societal norms.

This historical context of suppression and stigmatization forms a critical backdrop for our exploration of the recent resurgence of interest in psychedelics. Understanding the regulatory and societal shifts that occurred in the mid-20th century provides essential context for appreciating the challenges and opportunities faced by contemporary efforts to reevaluate the therapeutic potential of these substances.

Psychological Insights

Psychedelics can have a profound impact on the human psyche. These substances have the unique ability to facilitate introspection, dissolve ego boundaries, and bring repressed emotions to the surface. Clinical studies attest to their potential in treating a myriad of psychological issues, with a particular focus on their application in aiding combat veterans in their healing process.

Psychedelics, such as psilocybin and MDMA, have been shown to act as catalysts for introspection and self-reflection. These substances can help individuals explore their thoughts, emotions, and past experiences from differing perspectives, often leading to profound insights and personal growth.

One of the hallmark effects of psychedelics is the temporary dissolution of ego boundaries. This can result in a sense of unity with the universe or a profound interconnectedness with others and nature. For individuals burdened by the weight of trauma or emotional scars, this dissolution of ego can provide a fresh perspective and an opportunity to release deeply held pain.

Psychedelics have the capacity to unearth repressed emotions and memories, which can be particularly relevant in the context of trauma and PTSD. By bringing suppressed feelings to the surface, individuals have the chance to confront and process them, often leading to a reduction in symptoms associated with trauma.

Clinical studies have demonstrated the potential of psychedelic-assisted therapy in treating combat veterans with PTSD. Research with substances like MDMA has shown promising results in reducing symptoms and improving overall well-being. The healing process often involves revisiting traumatic memories with the support of a trained therapist in a safe and controlled setting.

Beyond PTSD, psychedelics hold promise in addressing moral injury, a complex psychological condition that often afflicts combat veterans. Moral injury arises from the profound moral dilemmas faced during military service. Psychedelic-assisted therapy offers a unique avenue for individuals to navigate these complex emotions and find a path toward healing and reconciliation.

Emerging research suggests that psychedelics can be valuable tools in the treatment of substance use disorders. They can help individuals confront the underlying causes of addiction, break the cycle of dependency, and foster a renewed sense of purpose and meaning.

Throughout this exploration, we emphasize the paramount importance of professional guidance in the use of psychedelics. These substances are not a panacea but rather powerful tools that require careful and expertly guided experiences. Trained therapists play a pivotal role in ensuring the safety and efficacy of psychedelic-assisted psychotherapy.

Empirical evidence and clinical studies illuminate psychedelics' capacity to aid combat veterans in confronting and healing from trauma, moral injury, and substance use disorders, always within the context of professional guidance and support.

Philosophical Contemplations

Western philosophy has a rich tradition of introspection and self-exploration. Philosophers like Socrates, Plato, and Descartes have posed questions about the nature of the self and the limitations of human understanding. Psychedelics, with their capacity to dissolve ego boundaries and facilitate deep introspection, align with this tradition.

Psychedelics challenge the notion of a fixed and separate self. They often induce experiences of ego dissolution, where the boundaries between the individual and the world blur or disappear entirely. This mirrors the philosophical exploration of the self as a dynamic and interconnected entity rather than a rigid construct.

Eastern philosophical traditions, such as Buddhism and Taoism, emphasize interconnectedness and the concept of oneness. Psychedelic experiences frequently align with these teachings by providing individuals with a direct, experiential understanding of the interconnected nature of all existence.

In Eastern philosophy, the dissolution of dualities—such as self and other, subject and object—is a central theme. Psychedelics often facilitate experiences where these dualities dissolve, leading individuals to a state of unity and interconnectedness with all that exists.

Psychedelics offer a unique opportunity to synthesize Western and Eastern philosophical perspectives. They invite individuals to question their assumptions about the self, reality, and consciousness, fostering a more holistic and integrative worldview.

Both Western and Eastern philosophies share a common aspiration for spiritual awakening and enlightenment. Psychedelics can serve as catalysts for these experiences, providing glimpses into states of consciousness that align with the highest aspirations of both traditions.

These philosophical contemplations have practical implications for individuals who seek personal growth and spiritual development. Psychedelic-assisted therapy can be viewed as a modern-day ritual or tool for achieving profound insights and transformation, guided by the wisdom of both Western and Eastern philosophies.

Veterans

As discussed in detail in Part I, combat veterans often grapple with moral injury, a profound psychological wound resulting from actions or witnessed events that violate deeply held moral beliefs and values. These experiences can leave enduring emotional scars and existential questions.

Moral injury is intertwined with existential questions about the nature of humanity, the consequences of one's actions, and the meaning of life itself. Combat veterans may find themselves haunted by these questions, struggling to reconcile their wartime experiences with their moral compass.

Psychedelics are catalysts and have shown remarkable potential in facilitating deep introspection and exploration of existential themes. They can help individuals confront the existential anguish associated with moral injury, providing a safe and supportive space for this exploration.

Moral injury often leads to overwhelming feelings of guilt and shame. Psychedelic experiences can assist individuals in confronting and processing these emotions, facilitating self-forgiveness and healing.

Psychedelics can guide combat veterans on a journey of self-compassion and self-understanding. By revisiting and reevaluating their wartime experiences, individuals may move toward acceptance and inner peace.

Through the lens of psychedelics, combat veterans can reconnect with their core values and beliefs. This reconnection may help them make sense of their moral injuries and find a renewed sense of purpose and meaning in life.

As always, it is essential to emphasize that the exploration of moral injury with psychedelics should be conducted under the guidance of trained therapists. Professional support ensures a safe and therapeutic context for these deeply transformative experiences.

Historical Perspectives

Throughout history, psychedelics have held a sacred and revered place in various cultures and spiritual traditions. From the use of psilocybin-containing mushrooms in ancient Mesoamerican rituals to the Ayahuasca ceremonies in the Amazon rainforest, these substances have been referred to as "sacred medicines." In these contexts, psychedelics were believed to open a direct channel to the divine and facilitate encounters with the numinous and the mystical.

Psychedelic experiences often transcend the ordinary and evoke a profound sense of the numinous—a feeling of awe and reverence in the presence of something greater than oneself. The dissolution of ego boundaries can lead to a direct and unfiltered connection with the sacred, bringing individuals face-to-face with the mysteries of existence.

Psychedelics have the remarkable capacity to induce mystical experiences characterized by a profound sense of unity, interconnectedness, and ineffability. Mystical experiences often involve a direct encounter with the divine or a sense of oneness with the cosmos. These encounters can be deeply transformative and provide individuals with a transcendent perspective on life.

In contemporary settings, the exploration of the spiritual dimensions of psychedelics has gained renewed interest. Researchers, therapists, and individuals seeking personal growth are increasingly recognizing the potential of these substances to facilitate profound spiritual experiences.

For combat veterans grappling with the complex aftermath of their service, the spiritual dimensions of psychedelic experiences can offer a sense of purpose and transcendence. These experiences may help individuals find meaning in their lives, reconcile their wartime experiences, and navigate the challenges of post-military existence.

The integration of spiritual insights gained from psychedelic experiences can be a critical part of the healing process. It involves making sense of the mystical and numinous encounters and incorporating their lessons into one's daily life. Trained therapists play a pivotal role in guiding individuals through this process.

The exploration of the sacred and profane with psychedelics is not about dogma or doctrine but rather a deeply personal and experiential journey. It can be a means to rekindle a sense of connection—with oneself, with others, and with the universe. In this way, psychedelics serve as powerful tools for veterans seeking to rediscover a sense of purpose and transcendence in the aftermath of their military service.

In recent years, there has been a remarkable resurgence of interest in the therapeutic potential of psychedelics. This resurgence has been driven, in part, by a growing body of promising clinical trials that have demonstrated the efficacy of psychedelics in treating mental health conditions.

Research with substances like MDMA, psilocybin, and ketamine has shown significant benefits in reducing symptoms of PTSD, depression, anxiety, and substance use disorders.

One of the most significant catalysts for this resurgence has been the experiences and advocacy of combat veterans. Many veterans who have struggled with the devastating effects of PTSD and related conditions have turned to psychedelics as a last resort when conventional treatments proved ineffective. Their stories of profound healing and transformation have resonated deeply with both the public and policymakers.

The need for alternative and more effective treatments for combat veterans with PTSD and related conditions cannot be overstated. Traditional therapies have often yielded limited results, leaving many veterans trapped in a cycle of suffering. Psychedelic-assisted therapy offers a fresh and innovative approach that addresses the root causes of their psychological wounds.

Combat veterans, along with organizations like the Multidisciplinary Association for Psychedelic Studies (MAPS), have played a pivotal role in advocating for research and policy changes surrounding psychedelics. Their efforts have helped raise awareness about the potential benefits of these substances and have contributed to a shift in public perception and policy.

Some combat veterans have participated in specialized retreats that incorporate psychedelics into a structured therapeutic setting. These retreats, often led by experienced therapists, provide a supportive environment for veterans to confront and heal from their trauma. These retreat experiences have further bolstered the case for the therapeutic use of psychedelics in veteran care.

Despite the promising results, there are still challenges to be overcome in fully integrating psychedelics into veteran care. Regulatory hurdles, stigma, and the need for further research are among the obstacles that must be addressed. However, the recent resurgence fueled by veterans' advocacy and experiences has set the stage for a new era in which psychedelics may play a vital role in healing psychological wounds.

CHAPTER 7

The Neuroscience of
Psychedelics

In the vast and complex theater of mental health, there exists a silent crisis: the enduring battle waged within the minds of combat veterans. Traditional therapies, while effective for some, often fall short for those scarred by the unseen wounds of war. Here, in the realm of synaptic interplays and neural pathways, lies the potential of an unconventional ally—psychedelic-assisted psychotherapy. This emergent paradigm, which once skirted the fringes of scientific inquiry, now shines as a beacon of hope for those grappling with the profound ramifications of post-traumatic stress disorder (PTSD), moral injury, and substance use disorders.

This chapter is a voyage into the cerebral cosmos, where the enigmatic actions of psychedelics reveal a compelling narrative of neuroplasticity and healing. We stand at the precipice of a new understanding, looking into the biochemical orchestration that unfolds when these substances interface with the brain's intricate circuitry. It honors the resilience of the human spirit and the boundless possibilities within the confluence of neurology and psychology.

As we embark on this journey, we aim to demystify the mechanisms by which these molecules impart their profound effects. From the serotonin pathways that they co-opt to the existential revelations they induce, psychedelics can redefine the mental landscapes of those who have navigated the darkest alleys of human experience. This chapter articulates how, by unlocking the mind's hidden potential, these compounds may facilitate a catharsis that conventional methods have yet to achieve.

By interlacing the latest scientific insights with the nuanced needs of combat veterans and their families, we will explore how psychedelics may recalibrate the traumatized brain. It is a narrative of transformation —how molecules become mediators of mind and how the essence of trauma can be re-envisioned through their use.

This exploration is not merely academic; it is a call to deepen our understanding and to compassionately apply our knowledge to the service of those who have endured the din of combat. In doing so, we recognize the gravity of the topic and the profound responsibility that accompanies using these powerful tools. With each page, we seek not only to inform but to evoke a sense of curiosity, hope, and reverence for the potential of psychedelic-assisted psychotherapy to offer a salve to the psyche and a bridge to a more serene state of being for our veterans and their loved ones.

How Psychedelics Affect the Brain

To comprehend the therapeutic potential of psychedelics, it is imperative to understand their physiological underpinnings. These compounds, often classified as serotonergic hallucinogens, exert their influence by interfacing with the serotonergic system—primarily by binding to the serotonin 2A receptor. Serotonin, a pivotal neurotransmitter in the modulation of mood and cognition, serves as a cornerstone for the psychedelics' multifaceted impact. This biochemical mimicry initiates a cascade of synaptic events, with effects that are as diverse as they are profound.

Psychedelics' effects are far-reaching within the cerebral landscape, but they cast a powerful influence over the prefrontal cortex, amygdala, and thalamus. The prefrontal cortex, which orchestrates our executive functions and moderates social behavior, is invigorated under the influence of these substances, potentially enhancing cognitive flexibility and creativity.

Meanwhile, the amygdala, the emotional sentinel of our brain, becomes more receptive to emotional stimuli. This increased emotional acuity can be a double-edged sword, intensifying emotional responses but also potentially providing therapeutic breakthroughs as veterans revisit traumatic memories in a new and often more manageable light.

The thalamus, a switchboard for sensory information, experiences a modulation of its gating mechanisms under psychedelics, which may lead to the sensory and perceptual alterations characteristic of the psychedelic experience. This can result in a more integrated and less filtered experience of the world, sometimes described by users as a sense of oneness or interconnectedness with their environment.

The 'entropic brain' theory posits that psychedelics induce a state of increased neural randomness, which can be quantified as increased entropy. Within controlled therapeutic contexts, this elevated entropy is not merely chaotic but can be a fertile ground for reorganization. It is akin to shaking a snow globe: while the flakes are suspended in turbulence, new patterns and pathways become possible. In the aftermath of trauma, the brain's networks can become rigid and pathological. Still, the introduction of psychedelics may loosen these fixed patterns, granting the mind the flexibility to escape from destructive cycles and embrace new narratives.

Moreover, neuroimaging studies suggest that psychedelics reduce activity in the default mode network (DMN), an interconnected group of brain regions that govern self-referential thought processes, including rumination. This quieting of the DMN correlates with the ego-dissolution and unitive experiences reported by individuals under the influence of these substances and may play a role in their potential to reframe self-centric narratives often associated with trauma and depression.

As this chapter unfolds, we will dissect the multifaceted effects of psychedelics with a focus on their transformative potential as chemicals and keys to unlocking the enigmatic doors within the human mind. Through a scientific lens, we will delve deeper into the intricacies of these substances, offering insights that are at once profound and grounded, reflective of the vast and still largely uncharted neural terrain they affect. The 'entropic brain' hypothesizes that psychedelics increase the brain's information entropy, allowing for an increase in neural connections and a breakdown of rigid thought patterns.

Benefits for Combat-Exposed Veterans

Combat-exposed veterans often return from service bearing the invisible but heavy armor of psychological distress. Traditional pharmacotherapies and psychotherapies sometimes falter under the weight of complex post-traumatic stress disorder (PTSD) symptoms, leaving veterans in search of alternative avenues for healing. Psychedelic-assisted psychotherapy is emerging as a potent catalyst for mental health transformation in this unique population.

The therapeutic benefits of psychedelics for combat-exposed veterans can be multifaceted. On a neural level, these substances may facilitate a 'neural reset,' where the rigid patterns of thought and memory, which are hallmarks of PTSD, become more malleable. This neural plasticity allows for the reevaluation and recontextualization of traumatic memories. When coupled with psychotherapy, psychedelics may help dislodge the cognitive and emotional impasses that contribute to symptoms like flashbacks, hypervigilance, and insomnia.

Psychedelics also appear to decrease the hyperactivity of the amygdala, a region that is often overactive in individuals with PTSD. This can reduce the immediate, visceral reactions to traumatic memories, granting veterans a level of emotional detachment that can be therapeutically beneficial. By dampening the fear response, psychedelics may facilitate a more tempered approach to trauma processing, enabling veterans to confront their experiences with reduced emotional turmoil.

The entropic effect on the brain produced by psychedelics is also noteworthy. In a controlled therapeutic setting, this increased entropy may allow veterans to break free from the persistent, intrusive thoughts that often characterize PTSD. There's a potential for psychedelics to catalyze profound epiphanies and insights, fostering a sense of connectedness and spiritual well-being that can be particularly restorative for those feeling disconnected from themselves and the world around them.

Furthermore, psychedelics may help in addressing moral injury—a form of psychological distress that occurs when one's actions, or the actions of others, transgress deeply held moral beliefs and expectations—that are frequently experienced by combat veterans. The introspective experiences promoted by psychedelics, within the safety of a therapeutic context, may offer opportunities for veterans to reconcile these moral conflicts, find forgiveness, and foster a greater sense of inner peace.

While these potential benefits are compelling, it is paramount to acknowledge and navigate the limitations and risks associated with psychedelic use. Appropriate screening, professional guidance, and a supportive setting are critical to harnessing the potential benefits while minimizing potential harm. This journey of healing is not a solo endeavor. As such, psychedelic-assisted therapy should be approached with the support of trained mental health professionals who can provide the necessary framework for a safe and transformative experience.

As research progresses, the promise of psychedelics as a tool for healing the minds of those who have served in combat continues to grow. The evidence suggests that, for many veterans, these substances may offer a chance to dampen the symptoms of PTSD and help to reengage with life in a more meaningful and peaceful way.

Specific Overviews – Benefits & Limitations

Psilocybin, a naturally occurring psychedelic compound found in certain species of mushrooms, has been the subject of revitalized research interest, especially for its therapeutic potential in treating mental health disorders. This section looks into the mechanism of action, medicinal and therapeutic value, and limitations of psilocybin, with a specific focus on its relevance to combat-exposed veterans.

Psilocybin primarily activates serotonin receptors in the brain, specifically the 5- HT2A receptor. Upon ingestion, psilocybin is converted into psilocin, its active form, which then profoundly impacts the brain's serotonergic system. Activating these receptors leads to altered consciousness and perception, often manifesting as a transcendental or mystical-like experience for the individual.

The psychedelic experience induced by psilocybin can lead to a temporary dissolution of the ego by inhibiting the Default Mode Network. Various researchers suggest this might be at the core of its therapeutic effects. This ego dissolution facilitates a state of increased psychological flexibility, which can be harnessed in therapeutic settings to restructure maladaptive thought patterns and emotional responses, especially those rooted in traumatic experiences.

For veterans, the therapeutic potential of psilocybin lies in its capacity to facilitate profound and often life-affirming insights. It has shown promise in alleviating chronic depression and anxiety, conditions that frequently co-occur with PTSD. The introspective journey psilocybin induces can provide a new perspective on past traumas, potentially leading to reconciliation and a newfound sense of peace.

Research has found that psilocybin-assisted therapy can significantly reduce symptoms of depression and anxiety for extended periods following just a single dose. This feature represents a considerable advantage over traditional antidepressants. Moreover, the transcendental experiences reported by many users can instill a sense of connectedness and unity, counteracting the isolating effects of PTSD and leading to a greater sense of purpose, connectivity, and overall well-being.

Despite its potential, psilocybin is not a universal remedy. Its use comes with limitations and is not suitable for everyone. Specific populations, including individuals with a history of psychosis or bipolar disorder, may be at increased risk for adverse reactions. Furthermore, the setting in which psilocybin is administered is crucial; an unsupportive or unpredictable environment can lead to very challenging experiences.

Integrating profound experiences into one's everyday life is also challenging. Without proper guidance and psychotherapeutic support, the insights gained during a psilocybin session may not translate into long-term change. Ensuring the presence of trained therapists before, during, and after the psychedelic experience is paramount to its success as a therapeutic tool.

Lastly, there are legal and regulatory limitations to consider. Psilocybin remains a Schedule I substance under federal law in many countries, significantly limiting its availability for therapeutic use and research. As policy evolves, so does the accessibility of psilocybin for those in need.

Psilocybin holds a unique place in the psychedelic pharmacopeia, offering profound therapeutic potential for combat-exposed veterans. Its ability to catalyze transformative experiences may unlock new pathways to healing. However, it must be approached carefully, considering its limitations, and under professional supervision to ensure the safety and well-being of those served.

MDMA, 3,4-methylenedioxymethamphetamine, commonly known as MDMA, has gained considerable attention in the context of psychotherapy for its unique psychopharmacological properties. Unlike traditional psychedelics such as LSD or psilocybin, MDMA is known primarily for its empathogenic effects. This section will explore MDMA's mechanism of action, its therapeutic potential, and its limitations in the treatment of veterans with combat-related psychological trauma.

MDMA's primary action is on the brain's serotonergic system, which influences dopamine and norepinephrine levels. It leads to the release of large amounts of serotonin, along with other neurotransmitters, which profoundly affect mood and perception. Crucially, MDMA also promotes the release of hormones such as oxytocin and prolactin, which play roles in social bonding and trust, enhancing the feeling of emotional closeness and empathy toward others.

The mechanism of action for MDMA is multifaceted. By increasing the release of serotonin, MDMA significantly impacts the amygdala, reducing the fear response and dampening the emotional impact of traumatic memories. This effect and increased oxytocin levels may lower defenses and promote a sense of safety and trust in therapeutic settings, thus facilitating deeper emotional processing.

MDMA's ability to foster empathy and reduce the fear response is particularly beneficial in psychotherapeutic settings for veterans who often face challenges with emotional connection and trust due to PTSD. The drug's effects can create an optimal psychological state for patients to engage in therapeutic work, potentially allowing them to address traumatic memories with reduced emotional pain and increased insight.

The trajectory of MDMA-assisted psychotherapy, especially in the context of treating PTSD in combat veterans, has been substantially informed by the structured clinical trials conducted by the Multidisciplinary Association for Psychedelic Studies (MAPS). The outcomes of these trials, spanning Phase 1, 2, and 3, have progressively solidified the therapeutic credentials of MDMA in clinical settings.

Initial Phase 1 clinical trials primarily focused on the safety profile of MDMA. These trials established a foundational understanding of the pharmacokinetics and pharmacodynamics of MDMA in the human body, confirming that, under controlled conditions, MDMA had an acceptable safety margin and warranted further investigation for therapeutic use.

Phase 2 trials began to explore the efficacy of MDMA-assisted psychotherapy while also building on safety data. These trials were pivotal in highlighting the drug's potential, with many participants experiencing significant reductions in PTSD symptoms. Phase 2 trials were diverse, involving various demographics, including combat veterans, first responders, and victims of sexual assault. The consistent theme across these studies was the enhancement of the therapeutic alliance— MDMA facilitated a level of rapport and trust between therapist and patient that became a catalyst for profound therapeutic engagement.

The Phase 3 trials marked a critical phase in the scientific validation of MDMA-assisted psychotherapy. As the final stage required for potential FDA approval, these trials were more significant in scale and sought to confirm the efficacy findings from Phase 2. The results were compelling; patients who received MDMA-assisted psychotherapy demonstrated significantly greater improvements in PTSD symptoms compared to those who received placebo, with over two-thirds of participants no longer qualifying for a PTSD diagnosis after just two sessions of MDMA-assisted psychotherapy. These trials underscored MDMA's ability to facilitate deep psychological work by promoting emotional openness and reducing fear and defensiveness during the processing of traumatic memories.

The impact of MDMA on the therapeutic alliance cannot be overstated. By fostering a sense of empathy and connection, MDMA helps create an environment where patients feel safe to expose and explore the most vulnerable facets of their psyche. This emotional safety net is particularly crucial for veterans, whose experiences often leave them isolated and guarded. The enhanced alliance facilitates emotional engagement and honest dialogue essential for effective psychotherapy, frequently leading to breakthroughs that might otherwise be unattainable or require a much more extended period through conventional therapy.

The MAPS-sponsored clinical trials have not only demonstrated the potential of MDMA as a powerful adjunct to psychotherapy but also paved the way for its consideration as a legitimate and regulated treatment option for those who have PTSD. The continued success of these trials is a precursor for the potential FDA approval and subsequent availability of MDMA- assisted psychotherapy for those in dire need of effective treatment options.

Despite its potential, MDMA-assisted therapy is not without limitations. The most pressing is the need for controlled settings and structured support to manage the intense emotions and altered state of consciousness induced by the drug. The potential for abuse and the adverse cardiovascular effects of MDMA necessitate careful screening of participants, as well as monitored administration by trained professionals.

The therapeutic effects of MDMA are not permanent and typically require integration sessions to help patients process their experiences and apply insights to their daily lives. Additionally, there can be side effects during the experience, such as anxiety, increased heart rate, or blood pressure, and these must be carefully managed.

There are also regulatory hurdles, as MDMA is classified as a Schedule I substance in many jurisdictions, reflecting high control and limited accepted medical use.

However, recent breakthrough therapy designations in some countries indicate changing perceptions and potential for more comprehensive therapeutic applications in the future.

The empathogenic qualities of MDMA represent a powerful adjunct to psychotherapy for veterans struggling with PTSD and related conditions. Its ability to enhance emotional processing and connection can catalyze therapeutic progress. However, it must be administered cautiously and within the boundaries of a structured therapeutic protocol to mitigate risks and optimize benefits.

Ketamine, historically utilized as an anesthetic, has gained considerable attention in recent years for its rapid-acting antidepressant properties. Its therapeutic application, particularly among combat veterans suffering from severe depression and suicidality, presents a new frontier in psychopharmacology.

Unlike traditional antidepressants that target the monoaminergic system, ketamine interacts with the glutamatergic system by antagonizing the N-methyl-D-aspartate (NMDA) receptor. This blockade increases glutamate, the most abundant excitatory neurotransmitter in the brain. The surge in glutamate triggers a cascade of events that lead to the release of growth factors and the formation of new synaptic connections, a process known as synaptogenesis.

Ketamine thus promotes neural plasticity, which can potentially rejuvenate neural circuits impaired by stress and depression.

The appeal of ketamine in a clinical setting lies in its ability to provide relief within hours, as opposed to the weeks or even months that conventional antidepressants may require. This rapid action can be life-saving for veterans grappling with acute suicidal ideation. Furthermore, ketamine's ability to help patients step outside of their entrenched thought patterns has been likened to 'chemical psychotherapy,' allowing for cognitive flexibility and the reframing of traumatic experiences during psychotherapeutic interventions.

Ketamine is administered in various forms, with intravenous infusions being the most studied in clinical trials. Other methods include intranasal sprays, like the FDA-approved Esketamine, oral tablets, and sublingual lozenges. Treatment protocols often involve a series of doses over a few weeks, combined with ongoing psychotherapy, to maximize therapeutic outcomes.

Despite its promise, ketamine's use comes with caveats. The dissociative effects, which can be therapeutic in a controlled environment, may be disorienting or distressing for some patients. There is also the risk of abuse and the potential for cognitive impairment with long-term use. Furthermore, the transient nature of ketamine's benefits means that without additional psychological support or repeat dosing, depressive symptoms can return.

Lastly, the heterogeneity of response in patients suggests that ketamine may not be universally effective. Future research is critical to elucidating which patients are most likely to benefit and how to maintain the antidepressant effects of ketamine over the long term with minimal risks.

Ketamine represents a profound shift in the treatment of refractory depression and PTSD among veterans, providing rapid relief and a novel therapeutic pathway. However, it demands careful consideration regarding its administration, potential side effects, and the structure of accompanying psychotherapeutic support.

Ibogaine is a psychoactive alkaloid derived from the root bark of the African shrub Tabernanthe iboga. Its complex pharmacological profile sets it apart as a substance with potential for treating addiction, which may particularly benefit veterans dealing with substance use disorders.

Ibogaine's mechanism is multifaceted, affecting several neurotransmitter systems. Primarily, it acts as a non-competitive antagonist at NMDA receptors and as an agonist at sigma-2 receptors, which may underlie its anti-addictive properties. Additionally, Ibogaine modulates opioid receptors and serotonin transporters, affecting mood and addiction patterns. Its metabolite noribogaine has a prolonged half-life and contributes to the lasting effects of Ibogaine by influencing the opioid system, which is often dysregulated in addiction.

The therapeutic potential of Ibogaine lies in its reported ability to alleviate withdrawal symptoms and reduce drug craving, thereby serving as a bridge to sobriety for individuals battling addiction. Veterans suffering from substance use disorders may find in Ibogaine a powerful ally that can interrupt the cycle of addiction, offering a window of clarity wherein therapeutic interventions can take root.

Some small-scale studies and anecdotal reports have suggested that Ibogaine can facilitate profound psychological insights and self-reflection, assisting individuals in confronting and reevaluating the emotional and psychological aspects of their addiction. This introspective journey may be particularly valuable for veterans who may have turned to substances as a coping mechanism for trauma or PTSD.

Despite its potential, Ibogaine's therapeutic use is limited by significant safety concerns. It can cause bradycardia ataxia and, in some instances, has been associated with life-threatening cardiac arrhythmias. Its safety profile necessitates close medical supervision when administered. Furthermore, the lack of large-scale, randomized controlled trials means that much of the evidence for Ibogaine's efficacy remains anecdotal or derived from observational studies with inherent limitations.

Legal barriers also restrict the use of Ibogaine, as it is classified as a Schedule I substance in the United States and is similarly controlled in many other countries. The need for further research is paramount to establish standardized dosing protocols, assess long-term outcomes, and fully understand the risks versus the benefits of its use in treating addiction.

Ibogaine represents a controversial yet potentially revolutionary approach to addiction treatment. Its capacity to disrupt addictive behaviors could offer significant relief for veterans struggling with substance dependence. However, the real-world application of ibogaine therapy requires a careful balance of its promising therapeutic effects against the real risks it poses, necessitating a thorough and cautious approach to its use.

DMT, Dimethyltryptamine, is a naturally occurring psychedelic compound of the tryptamine family; its presence is an enigma that spans various species of plants and the animal kingdom. Revered for its entheogenic use, DMT is found in an array of botanical sources, such as Psychotria viridis and Banisteriopsis caapi, which are central to the traditional Amazonian brew known as ayahuasca. In the animal kingdom, it is notably present in the secretions of the Colorado River toad, also known as the Bufo toad, offering a unique and potent variant known as 5-MeO-DMT. This molecule, sometimes called the "God Molecule," is sought after for its rapid and profound psychoactive effects, which have captivated the scientific community's interest and those seeking spiritual awakening. The enigmatic origins of DMT, bridging the gap between flora and fauna, set the stage for a deep dive into the complex interactions it fosters within the human brain.

Within the intricacies of life, DMT stands as a compound not only external to us but also as an intrinsic part of our biological makeup. Intriguingly, DMT is endogenously produced in the human body, with research suggesting its presence in the pineal gland, a small endocrine gland in the brain. It is hypothesized that this enigmatic molecule plays a role in near-death experiences, as it is believed to be released in significant amounts during the final moments of life, flooding the brain with its consciousness-altering effects. This natural occurrence of DMT within us speaks to a profound connection between the external forces of nature and our internal landscapes. This connection continues to mystify and inspire the scientific and spiritual communities alike.

The mechanism of action of 5-MeO-DMT is an opus of neurochemical activity that orchestrates a profound alteration in consciousness. To understand this mechanism, it is necessary to delve into the intricate workings of the brain's serotonergic system.

The serotonergic system, which relies on the neurotransmitter serotonin, plays a pivotal role in regulating mood, cognition, and perception. 5-MeO-DMT exerts its effects by binding to serotonin receptors, mimicking the action of serotonin itself. The most critical of these receptors for the psychedelic experience is the 5-HT2A receptor.

When 5-MeO-DMT binds to the 5-HT2A receptor, it triggers a conformational change in the receptor structure, setting off a cascade of intracellular events. These events involve different signaling pathways, such as the phospholipase C pathway, which releases calcium ions and activates protein kinase C.

This activation has a downstream effect on various neurotransmitter systems, including dopamine and glutamate. The alteration in dopamine levels can affect reward and pleasure centers, potentially providing therapeutic benefits for those experiencing anhedonia as part of depression or PTSD. The modulation of glutamate transmission affects neural plasticity—the brain's ability to change and adapt—which is essential for learning and memory.

Beyond individual neurotransmitters, 5-MeO-DMT disrupts the default mode network (DMN), a network of brain regions that is active during rest and self-referential thought processes. This disruption is associated with the experience of ego dissolution, where the sense of self is altered or temporarily lost, allowing for a sensation of unity and oneness with the environment. The DMN has been implicated in the maintenance of rigid patterns of thinking and behavior, such as those found in various mental health disorders, and its disruption may underlie the therapeutic potential of psychedelics.

5-MeO-DMT also induces a state of hyperconnectivity in the brain, where regions that do not typically communicate directly with each other begin to do so. This increased connectivity can lead to the unusual perceptions and synesthesia (cross-sensory experiences) often reported by users. It may also enable the brain to form new connections and perspectives, potentially contributing to lasting changes in outlook and behavior.

The ability of 5-MeO-DMT to induce plasticity and disrupt entrenched neural patterns is particularly relevant to its therapeutic potential. For combat veterans with PTSD, these effects could translate into a loosening of the rigid thought patterns associated with the disorder, enabling the processing and integration of traumatic memories.

However, the powerful effects of 5-MeO-DMT on brain chemistry also underscore its potential risks. The intensity of the experience can be psychologically challenging, necessitating careful screening, preparation, and support for those undergoing therapy. Moreover, the possibility of serotonin syndrome, a potentially life-threatening condition, underlines the need for professional oversight when using this compound therapeutically.

5-MeO-DMT's mechanism of action within the brain is multifaceted, involving receptor binding, neurotransmitter modulation, and network disruption. This intricate dance of neurochemical activity paves the way for its profound psychoactive effects, which can be harnessed for therapeutic benefit under the right conditions. The substance's capacity to prompt a reconfiguration of neural networks holds promise for the treatment of conditions characterized by maladaptive neural patterns, such as PTSD, offering the potential for healing and transformation for suffering combat veterans.

Lysergic acid diethylamide, more commonly known as LSD, is a synthetic psychedelic known for its powerful alteration of perception, emotions, and the sense of time. The following section will provide a comprehensive look into the benefits and limitations of LSD, particularly in the context of therapeutic applications for long-term trauma.

LSD exerts its effects primarily by interacting with serotonin receptors in the brain, especially the 5-HT2A receptor. Upon binding to these receptors, LSD initiates a complex signaling cascade that leads to changes in brain chemistry and cognition. Unlike other serotonergic psychedelics, LSD has a unique property known as 'functional selectivity' that allows it to have different effects on various types of cells, which could explain some of the unique characteristics of an LSD experience.

The compound's impact extends beyond the serotonin system. It affects the glutamate pathways, crucial for synaptic plasticity—the brain's ability to change and adapt. LSD also modulates the brain's dopamine systems, influencing motivation, drive, and reward experience. This broad spectrum of interaction within the brain's neurochemistry is what gives LSD its potent psychoactive capabilities.

The therapeutic benefits of LSD have been explored in various contexts, from its potential to treat alcoholism to its use in alleviating end-of-life anxiety. Its capacity to induce psychological flexibility is of particular interest. Psychological flexibility is a state where individuals are more open to new experiences, able to break free from rigid patterns of thought and behavior, and can reinterpret traumatic memories from a different perspective.

For combat veterans and individuals with long-term trauma, this psychological flexibility can manifest as an increased openness to therapeutic interventions, allowing for a reprocessing of traumatic events and a reduction in symptoms of disorders like PTSD. The altered state of consciousness induced by LSD can also lead to a sense of unity and connectedness, which can be profoundly transformative on a personal level.

However, the therapeutic use of LSD is not without its limitations. The duration of its effects— often lasting up to 12 hours—can be mentally and physically exhausting and may not be suitable for all individuals. The intensity and unpredictability of the experience also require a controlled environment and professional supervision to ensure safety and to navigate any challenging emotional or psychological terrain that may arise.

Additionally, LSD can interact with various medications and underlying health conditions, which must be carefully assessed before considering its use. The legal status of LSD, classified as a Schedule I substance in many parts of the world, further complicates its integration into mainstream therapeutic practices.

LSD presents a complex array of therapeutic potentials and challenges. Its ability to induce a state of psychological flexibility could provide significant benefits for those grappling with long-term trauma. Yet, it requires an approach considering the individual's psychological makeup, medical history, and legal landscape. While the horizon for clinical use of LSD is expanding, it remains a path that must be tread with caution, respect, and professional guidance.

Peyote, a cactus known scientifically as Lophophora williamsii, has been used for centuries in Native American spiritual traditions due to its psychoactive properties, primarily attributed to the compound mescaline. Its use in sacred rituals underscores a deep cultural and spiritual connection to healing and consciousness exploration. This section will provide a comprehensive look at the benefits and limitations of peyote within the context of therapeutic applications, especially in treating trauma.

Mechanism of Action: Mescaline, the primary active psychoactive compound in peyote, functions as a phenethylamine alkaloid with a similar structure to the neurotransmitter dopamine. It exerts its effects by binding to and activating serotonin receptors in the brain, particularly the 5-HT2A receptor, similar to other classical psychedelics. This receptor activation leads to an altered state of consciousness characterized by visual hallucinations, altered thought processes, and profound changes in perception and mood.

How It Works in the Brain: Mescaline's interaction with the serotonin system promotes increased neural connectivity and a breakdown of the normal hierarchies of brain function. This can lead to a disruption of the Default Mode Network (DMN), which is thought to play a role in self-referential thoughts and ego maintenance. By disrupting the DMN, mescaline may reduce the rigidity of established thought patterns and provide a mental environment where deeply ingrained traumas can be processed from a new perspective.

Therapeutic Value: The therapeutic value of peyote is found in its capacity to engender a profound psychological and spiritual experience, which can be particularly potent in a ritualistic or ceremonial setting. For those dealing with trauma, the introspective journey facilitated by peyote can offer a different view of past experiences, enabling individuals to confront and integrate their trauma with greater clarity and understanding.

Additionally, the sense of connectedness to a larger community or universe often experienced with peyote can help combat the feelings of isolation that often accompany trauma. This can be particularly meaningful for combat veterans who may feel disconnected from civilian life and are seeking a sense of belonging or purpose.

Limitations: Despite its potential benefits, the use of peyote also presents limitations. The psychoactive experience can be intense and may not be suitable for all individuals, especially those with a predisposition to psychotic disorders. The physical effects of mescaline, such as nausea and increased heart rate, can also be uncomfortable and pose risks to individuals with certain health conditions.

The legal status of peyote is complex. While it is a Schedule I controlled substance in the United States, there are exemptions for its use in religious ceremonies by the Native American Church. This legal framework can limit access to peyote for therapeutic use and complicate the integration of its benefits into more conventional medical practices.

Furthermore, the cultural significance of peyote must be approached with respect and sensitivity. Appropriation of Native American rituals and practices can be harmful and disrespectful, so it is crucial that the therapeutic use of peyote, when considered, is done in a manner that honors its sacred origins.

Peyote holds potential as a therapeutic agent for trauma, especially when its use is embedded within a framework of cultural reverence and spiritual significance. Its ability to facilitate deep introspection and a sense of unity makes it a unique tool in the healing journey. However, its application in therapy must be carefully managed, respecting both the individual's psychological state and the cultural dimensions of its use. As with all psychedelic substances, the promise of peyote comes with a need for careful consideration of its powerful effects, both positive and challenging.

Synergistic Effects of Ibogaine and 5-MeO-DMT

When considering the combined therapeutic use of Ibogaine and 5-MeO-DMT, it is vital to understand the specific interactions and synergistic effects that may occur because of their concurrent administration.

The pharmacological action of Ibogaine is multifaceted, affecting several brain regions and neurotransmitter systems that are implicated in addiction and mood disorders. Its metabolite, noribogaine, has a long duration of action, which extends its influence on the brain. On the other hand, 5-MeO-DMT exerts powerful psychoactive effects through its action on the serotonin receptors, particularly the 5-HT2A subtype.

When used in conjunction, Ibogaine may prime the brain by enhancing neuroplasticity, thus making the mind more amenable to the effects of 5-MeO-DMT. The result could be a potentiated response to 5-MeO-DMT, characterized by profound introspection and mystical-type experiences. This may lead to a significant therapeutic effect as patients potentially gain deep personal insights and emotional catharsis.

In a controlled medical setting, combining these two substances could be engineered to optimize the window of heightened neuroplasticity induced by Ibogaine with the peak experiential effects of 5-MeO-DMT. This synergy may foster an environment where combat veterans can reprocess traumatic memories and reformulate their relationship with past experiences in a way that single substance sessions might not facilitate.

Theoretically, Ibogaine's introspective journey can help patients uncover the psychological roots of their trauma or addiction. Followed by the ego-dissolving effects of 5-MeO-DMT, this could lead to a reintegration of self and a profound sense of peace or resolution, which are often elusive in traditional therapeutic settings.

While the potential for therapeutic breakthroughs is significant, so too are the safety concerns when combining potent psychoactive substances. The combined use of Ibogaine and 5-MeO- DMT could exacerbate cardiovascular strain or precipitate psychiatric complications. In a controlled medical environment, stringent screening processes, close monitoring of vital signs, and immediate medical intervention capabilities are non-negotiable prerequisites.

Additionally, the psychological intensity of the experiences warrants a comprehensive support structure, including pre-session preparation and post-session integration therapy, to help veterans understand and assimilate their experiences into their ongoing recovery process.

Given the experimental nature of this combination, ethical considerations are paramount. Informed consent is critical, with clear communication of the potential risks and uncharted aspects of this therapeutic approach. From a legal standpoint, the substances in question may fall under regulatory restrictions, requiring a sanctioned medical or research context for their use.

The concurrent use of Ibogaine and 5-MeO-DMT holds significant promise in controlled medical settings, offering a new potential avenue for healing and recovery for combat veterans with PTSD or substance use disorders. However, the approach is experimental and requires careful consideration of the balance between potential benefits and risks. Ongoing research, clinical trials, and the development of comprehensive treatment protocols will be critical in establishing the efficacy and safety of this avant-garde therapeutic option.

***

As we stand on the cusp of a new era in psychotherapeutic interventions for combat veterans, we must remain grounded in the empirical rigor that forms the cornerstone of scientific inquiry.

Psychedelics, in the context of this discussion, are not presented as a panacea but as a significant tool in the therapeutic armory—one that could potentially lead many on a transformative journey toward healing.

The path to recovery for veterans suffering from the invisible wounds of war is arduous and complex. Psychedelic substances like Ibogaine and 5-MeO-DMT, particularly in combination, represent a beacon of hope, yet they also demand a cautious and evidence-based approach.

The anecdotal promise of these compounds must be carefully weighed against systematic research to ensure safety and efficacy.

As researchers and clinicians continue to explore the profound effects of psychedelics on the mind and spirit, it is our collective responsibility to ensure that this exploration is conducted with integrity, caution, and a deep respect for those who have served. The therapeutic potential of psychedelics is a harbinger of hope. This hope must be nurtured by the rigorous application of science and an unwavering commitment to the health and well-being of our veterans.

It is the disciplined application of psychedelic-assisted therapy that holds the key to unlocking the full spectrum of their therapeutic promise. For combat veterans and their families, this represents more than just a treatment—it is a potential passage to peace, a voyage to the very core of their being, and a chance to reclaim a life of purpose and connection. As science advances, so does the possibility of restoration and renewal for those who have borne the battle, their caregivers, and their communities.

PART III

Psychedelic Therapy:
An Alternative Avenue

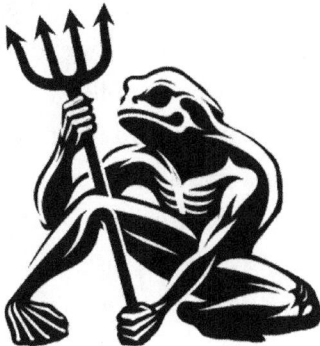

CHAPTER 8

A Synergetic Approach to Psychedelic Preparation

The path to healing from the scars of combat is as profound and complex as the human psyche itself. For veterans embarking on the journey of psychedelic-assisted psychotherapy, preparation is as crucial as the experience. This chapter is a compass for that preparation, with every word crafted to respect and understand the intricacies of a veteran's experience and the pivotal role of their families.

For Veterans: Education and Planning

Educate Yourself: The voyage into the realm of psychedelics is anchored in knowledge. This book serves as a repository of wisdom, offering a deep dive into the multifaceted effects, therapeutic potential, and possible risks associated with psychedelic substances. By engaging with the research and experiences compiled here, you are armed against misconceptions and pave a path toward informed decisions.

This book, therefore, is a preparation companion and a tool to help calibrate your expectations. It is also a map that points to the waypoints of careful, conscientious psychedelic use. As you turn each page, let it fortify your resolve and illuminate your path, ensuring that when you embark on this transformative journey, you do so with the utmost confidence and clarity.

Strategic Planning: Precision and strategy, hallmarks of military operations, are crucial in preparing for a psychedelic journey. This book outlines how to methodically select the right professionals—those who grasp the nuances of a veteran's experience—and how to tailor the psychedelic approach to your specific needs.

Consider this a strategic manual for planning your journey: identifying the right team, understanding legal considerations, and arranging the therapeutic setting. The focus and discipline you've honed during service are now pivotal in navigating this new terrain toward healing.

For Families: Understanding and Support

Gaining Insight: Your supportive journey is as vital as your veteran's individual quest for healing. Your comprehension of psychedelic therapy's subtleties becomes the beacon that lights their way and the foundation on which their healing process builds. This book dedicates itself to offering you a thorough education on what psychedelic therapy entails, going beyond mere definitions to explore its profound implications on mental health, particularly for those who have faced the crucibles of combat.

As you delve into these chapters, you'll gain a nuanced understanding of how psychedelics can catalyze healing, the importance of set and setting, and the potential for profound transformation. This insight will equip you to be an informed and compassionate ally. It will enable you to engage in meaningful conversations with your veteran, ask insightful questions of healthcare providers, and provide a level of knowledgeable and empathetic support.

Emotional and Logistical Support: Supporting a loved one through psychedelic therapy involves traversing an emotional landscape that may be as foreign to you as it is to the veteran that you love. Your ability to provide emotional support will be tested and strengthened as you learn to hold space for the vast spectrum of feelings and revelations that can emerge. This book offers guidance on how to be present for these moments, listen actively, respond with sensitivity, and maintain a supportive presence that respects the veteran's autonomy and journey.

Logistical support is equally crucial. It encompasses the practical aspects of preparing for the psychedelic sessions—from ensuring legal compliance and understanding the therapeutic protocols to managing the day-to-day tasks that may become secondary for a veteran deeply engaged in their healing work. You'll find practical advice on creating a serene and safe environment for the veteran, both during and after the therapy sessions, and tips on managing your own schedule and responsibilities to be as available as possible.

As families, your support system itself may need bolstering. This guide will also touch upon how to find and create a network of support for yourself, recognizing that in supporting a veteran, you, too, are embarking on a demanding and potentially transformative journey. It's a journey of learning, patience, and profound love that can be as healing for you as it is for the veteran you stand beside.

Preparing for the Psychedelic Journey

Setting Intentions: Intention-setting is a potent practice that steers the course of the psychedelic journey. Veterans stand to benefit by clearly defining their purpose for engaging with psychedelics, which could range from healing from trauma to reestablishing a sense of identity.

Family members support this process by facilitating open dialogue that helps veterans express their intentions. A therapist's expertise is invaluable here, providing a professional perspective that can help deepen the understanding of these intentions and how they can be manifested during the psychedelic experience.

This section will include strategies to set intentions effectively, with therapeutic exercises such as writing reflective letters, creating vision boards, or engaging in heartfelt conversations that bring to light the veteran's innermost hopes for the therapy.

Mental and Emotional Readiness Supported by Therapy: Mental and emotional preparedness is the foundation of a meaningful psychedelic experience. This readiness entails the courage to face and process complex emotions and past traumas. Veterans may connect with psychological theories that mirror their own journey—concepts like resilience and post-traumatic growth—that can be therapeutic in themselves. Here, therapists can play a key role in introducing and integrating these theories into the preparation process, providing veterans and their families with a framework for understanding and growth.

Included will be guidance on how therapeutic practices, such as meditation and mindfulness, can be adopted by both veterans and their families, creating a united front of healing and emotional readiness.

Physical and Spiritual Preparation with a Therapist's Touch: The synergy between physical well-being and psychological health is critical, especially in preparation for psychedelic therapy. Therapists can offer advice on physical preparations, suggesting dietary changes and exercise routines that complement the emotional work. On the spiritual front, therapists can help explore and integrate personal beliefs and values, which is often a significant aspect of the psychedelic experience. This book will provide insights into how therapy can merge physical and spiritual readiness, ensuring that veterans and their families approach the session feeling centered and whole.

Creating a Supportive Environment with Professional Advice: The setting in which the psychedelic session unfolds is pivotal to its success. Therapists can lend their experience and help families create a safe and serene environment conducive to healing. We will offer practical tips on arranging a space with considerations for comfort, safety, and emotional resonance, ensuring the environment supports the veteran's journey.

Navigating Relationship Dynamics with Therapeutic Insight: Effective communication and boundary-setting are critical in the lead-up to, during, and after the psychedelic experience. This book will discuss how therapists can provide tools for enhancing communication, fostering empathy, and establishing healthy boundaries. These skills are essential for maintaining a balance of support and independence, allowing both veterans and their families to feel connected yet not overwhelmed.

Incorporating a therapist into each step of the preparation process ensures that veterans and their families are ready to embark on the journey with the guidance and support needed to navigate the complexities of a psychedelic experience. This comprehensive approach lays a foundation for a healing, collaborative, and transformative journey for all involved.

Veterans

> *Educate Yourself:* Engage deeply with credible sources to understand the potential effects and risks of psychedelics.

> *Set Intentions:* Clearly define what you hope to achieve through the therapy to guide your experience.

> *Engage in Pre-Therapy Sessions:* Participate in sessions with a qualified therapist to build a foundation of trust and understanding.

> *Health Check*: Ensure a complete medical evaluation is done to assess suitability for psychedelic therapy.

> *Mental Preparation*: Utilize mindfulness or other grounding techniques to prepare mentally for the experience.

> *Take the Necessary Time*: Embrace the thorough preparation process, understanding its critical role in your healing journey.

> *Maintain an Open Mind:* Approach the therapy openly, allowing the experience to unfold naturally without preset expectations.

> *Stay Connected*: Maintain and seek out supportive relationships with friends and family who can be pillars of strength throughout your experience.

Seek Professional Guidance: Regularly consult with healthcare professionals to ensure your therapy is well-informed and safe.

ShareYourHistory: Openly communicate your mental health background with your therapist to enable tailored and effective care.

For Supportive Family Members

Be Informed: Learn about psychedelic therapy to provide informed support.

Listen Actively: Empathize with your veteran family member's feelings and concerns.

Encourage Professional Support: Motivate the veteran to seek and maintain contact with professional help.

Self-Care: Take care of your mental and emotional health to be a stable support system.

Respect Boundaries: Understand and respect the veteran's need for space or silence as they prepare for therapy.

Honor the Experience: Fully recognize and respect the depth of the veteran's experience and the commitment required for the therapeutic process.

Support the Veteran's Autonomy: Encourage the veteran to define their own therapeutic objectives, supporting their journey without imposing your personal expectations.

Be Vigilant and Responsive: Stay alert to any signs of discomfort or reluctance from the veteran and take immediate action to address these concerns compassionately.

Embrace the Entire Journey: Understand that preparation is the foundation for a longer healing process and commit to being there every step of the way.

Validate and Explore Concerns: Approach the veteran's concerns with sincerity and encourage open communication with the therapy provider to ensure they are addressed adequately.

A Synergetic Approach to Psychedelic Preparation

In Chapter 8, we traverse the multifaceted landscape of preparation for psychedelic-assisted psychotherapy. We understand that for combat veterans, the wounds of war are physical and deeply psychological, and their healing requires a journey as profound as the psyche itself. The preparation stage is a preliminary and fundamental part of the therapeutic process. This chapter serves as a guide, a strategic manual, and a companion for veterans and their families as they navigate this terrain.

For veterans, education is the keystone. Armed with knowledge, they can approach their psychedelic journey with confidence and clarity, utilizing the precision and strategy reminiscent of their military training to select the right professionals and tailor the psychedelic approach to their individual needs.

Families of veterans play an equally crucial role. By gaining insight into the therapy and creating a supportive environment, they become integral to the healing process. We discussed the importance of staying connected, validating experiences, and maintaining open communication as they accompany their loved ones on this path.

To encapsulate the essence of preparation, we have distilled a list of dos that illuminate the importance of timing, openness, support, and continuity of care for veterans, as well as the unwavering support, empathy, and understanding needed from their families. It is about embracing the journey with all its intricacies and fostering a partnership between the veteran, their family, and the therapist.

As we conclude this chapter, we underscore the synergy between knowledge and emotional readiness, physical and spiritual harmony, and the nurturing of relationship dynamics. With the therapeutic guidance interwoven throughout the preparation process, veterans and their families are preparing for a session and laying the groundwork for a collaborative and profound transformative healing journey.

This chapter has prepared the ground for what lies ahead, ensuring that both veterans and their families step into the world of psychedelic-assisted psychotherapy with their eyes open to the challenges and their hearts ready for the possibilities of growth and healing.

CHAPTER 9

Veterans and Psychedelic Therapy

Psychedelic therapy, poised at the vanguard of psychiatric innovation, beckons a new era of healing for combat veterans. It is a confluence of age-old wisdom and cutting-edge science, providing fresh avenues for those grappling with the specters of war-induced trauma. This chapter delves deeper into the empirical studies and personal accounts that underscore the efficacy and transformative potential of psychedelic therapy for veterans.

The re-emergence of psychedelic therapy in the contemporary medical canon does not occur in a vacuum. It results from meticulous research and an evolving understanding of psychiatric care. The empirical studies exploring this therapeutic frontier reveal a consistent theme: profound psychological relief for veterans who have often found themselves at an impasse with traditional treatment modalities. These narratives of healing and transformation are not just clinical case points but beacons of hope, illuminating the path for fellow warriors in the shadow of psychological distress.

The empirical literature is replete with case studies that offer a window into the healing journeys of combat veterans. For instance, a qualitative study conducted on veterans undergoing MDMA-assisted psychotherapy highlighted remarkable reductions in PTSD symptoms, alongside increased feelings of self-compassion and interpersonal connection. Such case studies often emphasize the symptomatic relief and the profound existential and spiritual awakenings that can accompany these experiences.

Psychedelic therapy's therapeutic mechanisms are a braiding of psychological, neurobiological, and spiritual strands. Under vigilant professional guidance, these substances act as catalysts for the mind's intrinsic healing capabilities. They facilitate a profound re-examination and re-contextualization of traumatic memories, empowering veterans with a renewed sense of agency and purpose. This reclamation of self can be the cornerstone of a veteran's journey to reclaim their life from the clutches of trauma and substance dependency.

The concept of 'set and setting' is pivotal to the success of psychedelic therapy. The 'set' refers to the psychological attitude and preparation of the individual. In contrast, 'setting' refers to the physical and social environment in which the therapy occurs. Veterans often highlight the importance of the supportive and structured nature of the therapeutic setting in their recovery process. In such sanctuaries, they can bravely face their traumatic memories and reframe them into narratives of survival and growth.

In the quest for wholeness, psychedelic therapy does not limit itself to the confines of Western medicine. Incorporating Eastern meditative practices fosters a therapeutic milieu that honors the totality of the human experience. This integrative approach resonates with veterans, whose experiences often leave them seeking a reconnection to self, others, and the larger spectrum of life.

As we await the personal accounts of veterans who have walked this path, we ground our discussion in the robust body of empirical work that supports the potential of psychedelic therapy. The research underscores the potential and possibility for those who have served, suggesting that the next chapter in their lives can be one of peace and reconnection.

CHAPTER 10

Embracing the Psychedelic Journey

Preparing for the Descent

As you stand on the precipice of a new journey, one not measured by land traversed but by the depths of the psyche explored, it's essential to recognize the strength that has brought you here. All the life experiences, the grueling training, and the survival instincts honed during combat are your past trials and the very tools that have equipped you for this moment. "You've got this" is not just an affirmation; it's a fact, underscored by your history and the resilience it has forged within you.

The step you are about to take is one of courage, a leap into the depths of your mind where you will encounter a terrain as demanding as any you have known. Yet, just as you have worn your armor into battle, you come to this experience fortified by preparation and purpose. Your military training, which taught you discipline and the ability to remain calm under pressure, will serve you well as you embark on this psychedelic journey.

Remember, the medication you will soon ingest is a catalyst, one that will unlock doors within your mind, but it is your will and readiness to engage that will guide you through them. This is not a battle to fight but an experience to be welcomed with the same bravery that has defined your life.

At this stage, you've worked extensively with your therapist to understand your intentions and to build a mental framework for the experience. You've trained just as rigorously for this as any mission. Now, as you sit with the medication in hand, it's time to let go of expectations to free yourself from the desire to predict or control what comes next. Trust in the process, in the safety net woven by the presence of professionals and the intentions you've set.

Let your breath be your anchor, your heart be your guide, and your trained capacity for mindfulness be your compass. Ingest the medication with a commitment to be present, allow, and open yourself to the full spectrum of sensations and insights that will arise. There's no need to hold on tight; you can navigate this inner landscape just as you've traversed uncertain terrains.

In this chapter of your life, you are both the explorer and the map-maker. The intensity of emotions and the vividness of the mindscapes you'll encounter may challenge you, but they will not overwhelm you. Because you've faced challenges before—you've stared down adversity and emerged with a spirit tempered like steel.

So, as the effects begin, as the fabric of reality takes on new colors and dimensions, remember that you've trained for uncertainty. Every trial you've faced, and every obstacle you've overcome has led to this point of inner exploration.

You're not just ready—you are made for this. This is not an ordeal; it's an odyssey. An odyssey that does not ask for the formidable warrior alone but calls upon the wise, the curious, the seeker of truths that you have also become.

As the medication takes effect and the journey inward commences, let this mantra be your grounding force: "I've got this." Because you do, with every breath and beat of your heart, you are stepping into a space of healing and discovery—a journey as significant as any you've undertaken. Welcome to the path within, warrior. Your new battle, a battle for peace and understanding, begins now.

The Practice of Letting Go

In the realm of psychedelics, the art of letting go is more than a mere suggestion—it is a gateway to transcendence, a path to unity with the broader aspects of existence, which is echoed in transpersonal psychology. This psychological approach transcends the individual ego and taps into collective, spiritual, and metaphysical dimensions of the self. For you, warrior of both the tangible and intangible battlegrounds, this surrender is not a sign of defeat but an active engagement with a broader reality.

With its deep roots in mindfulness and acceptance, Buddhist psychology holds that our suffering arises from attachment—to desires, expectations, and outcomes. In your military training, you have been taught to maintain an unwavering focus, a form of attachment necessary for survival. Yet, in this journey, you are called to integrate the wisdom of Buddhism—seeing the attachment for what it is, a potential source of suffering, and learning to let go with intention and grace.

The process of letting go becomes a courageous act of trust, akin to the trust you placed in your squad and your training. It asks you to trust not in the solidity of the ground beneath your feet but in the fluidity of your consciousness. It's a trust that you are exactly where you need to be despite the absence of a discernible enemy or a clear mission.

You do not become passive by releasing expectations and outcomes; instead, you open yourself to the full spectrum of experiences without preconceived limits. It resembles the Zen concept of Shoshin, or "beginner's mind," where openness, eagerness, and lack of preconceptions allow for richer experiences.

By applying the lens of these psychological and spiritual frameworks, the psychedelic experience becomes a vessel for exploring the mind's limitless capacities. You become a warrior in a different sense—one who combats the inner clinging that hinders enlightenment and true freedom. The act of letting go is thus transformed into an active engagement with the present moment. It is a profound alignment with the here and now, where each thought, sensation, and emotion is observed, acknowledged, and released without judgment or attachment.

As you embark on this phase of your journey, you carry the legacy of your military service and the collective wisdom of centuries of contemplative practice. The expectation is no longer about controlling the external chaos but finding serenity within the internal vastness. The outcome is not to conquer but to liberate and uncover the interconnectedness of all things, including the depths of your psyche.

In the therapeutic setting, as the medicine begins its work, you are not only the observer but also the observed, the healer, as well as the healed. You realize that in letting go, you are not losing anything but are being given an opportunity to gain everything—insight, healing, and a profound understanding of the self that is both personal and transpersonal. As the borders of ego begin to soften under the influence of psychedelics, the river of your consciousness, once narrowly channeled by the banks of identity and story, now flows into the expansive sea of collective being.

In this confluence, your ability to let go becomes your greatest strength. It is a strength that lies not in the hands that once wielded weapons but in the heart that now seeks peace and in the mind that recognizes its boundless nature.

And so, you continue, warrior—equipped with a new armory composed of mindfulness, acceptance, and the eternal wisdom of letting go. Here, in the vast landscape of your inner world, you embody courage—a courage that whispers but resonates through the entirety of your being: "Let go..."

The Uncharted Mind: Embracing the Unknown with Inquisitive Valor

Embarking on a psychedelic journey is an invitation into the unexplored territories of the psyche, a provocation to pierce the veil that shrouds the deepest recesses of our consciousness. This journey, akin to the deployments you've known, asks you to confront the unknown—not with trepidation, but with the ignited spirit of discovery.

The unfolding of the unknown is not something to be feared but an exploration of curiosity and excitement. It is a reminder that beyond the veil lies a vast expanse rich with the potential for profound understanding. The unknown does not wish to be feared; it desires to be known, to reveal its secrets to those courageous enough to inquire.

Within the therapeutic space, as the molecules of the medicine begin to interact with the fabric of your mind, the veil lifts, and what was once concealed begins to clarify. With each breath and moment of mindful presence, you are not dissolving into the abyss but expanding into the vastness of your being.

When you allow curiosity to steer you, the unknown transforms. It becomes an invitation to an adventure, a provocation that ignites a yearning to delve into the uncharted aspects of the self. It beckons you with the promise of insights yet uncovered, wisdom yet untapped. Once daunting, the caverns of the mind now seem inviting; each shadow cast by the interplay of your inner light and darkness creates a nuanced understanding of your narrative.

The promise of exploration is clear: if you are willing to traverse these inner landscapes, you will find answers—perhaps not the ones you expected, but the ones you need. With the willingness to let go of the moorings of preconceived notions, clarity emerges, not as a sudden epiphany but as a gradual dawning, a serene acceptance of the vast complexity of your experience.

As you move through the psychedelically-induced introspection, you learn that allowing and accepting are not passive acts but intensely active engagements with your inner world that enable the consciousness to expand beyond the familiar shores of the ego. To take on this challenge is to take the hand of your experiences, no matter how difficult, and dance with them, learning their rhythm and wisdom.

It is the alchemy of the mind that psychedelics can catalyze—the transformation of fear into curiosity, confusion into clarity, and pain into wisdom. It is a process that does not diminish the reality of your past struggles but reframes them, offering a lens through which every observed experience is valuable within the context of life.

As a combat veteran, you have faced the unknown countless times, each instance fortifying your resilience and strength. You are encouraged to turn that courage inward and apply the same resilience to exploring your inner self. The psychedelic experience is your new mission, not defined by external coordinates but by the internal compass of curiosity.

Let this be your mantra as the unknown unfolds: "In my willingness to explore, I find answers. In my willingness to let go, I find clarity. In my willingness to allow and accept, I find wisdom." With these truths as your guide, venture forth into the vast, intricate world within, for it is there that the most significant discoveries about who you are and what you can become lie in wait.

The Safety Net

In the theater of war, although often feeling alone, soldiers face their trials with a myriad of support that extends from themselves outward through the entire US military. Similarly, in the theater of the mind that you enter with psychedelics, the notion of support is revolutionized.

Here, you are enveloped in a collective embrace, a safety net woven with the expertise and empathy of those accompanying you on this inward odyssey.

Your support team—composed of therapists specialized in psychedelic-assisted psychotherapy, guides trained in facilitating these profound journeys, and perhaps fellow veterans who share the silent knowledge of service, will be your community of care. These individuals are not mere bystanders but active participants in your journey, the guardians of your psychological and emotional well-being.

Their presence is a constant, a bulwark against the tumult of the experience. As you navigate through the waves of intense emotions and memories that may arise, their steadfast presence is the anchor. This anchor does not keep you from exploring the depths; it ensures you can dive deep without losing your way to the surface.

The safety net they provide is multi-layered, ensuring that every aspect of your experience is held with importance. It is in the compassionate gaze of the therapist, the gentle guidance of the facilitator, and the knowing nods of peers that you find a multidimensional support system.

This network is attuned to the gravity of your journey, recognizing the courage it takes to confront the psyche's enigmatic realms. They are the silent watchers of your bravery, the honored keepers of your trust, and gentle guides to the present moment when the journey traverses darker paths or higher planes of thought and feeling.

Within this cocoon of security, every emotion and every memory that cascades through you is allowed and accepted. You are encouraged to let these experiences flow so that you can witness them with the curiosity and courage you possess while knowing that the safety net is ever-present.

Their role is not to steer your journey but to ensure that you feel the freedom to explore, knowing they are there, a lifeline to which you can always return. This assurance is spoken—a palpable presence, a felt sense that imbues the space around you. It is a reminder that, although the journey is yours alone to traverse, the experience of healing is a collective endeavor.

As you move through each phase of the psychedelic experience, from the anticipation of ingestion to the unfolding of the subconscious mind, remember this net is finely tuned to your needs. It is responsive, adaptive, and, most importantly, rooted in a deep understanding of the unique landscapes you navigate as a combat veteran.

Allow yourself to lean into this net when needed, to use it as a touchstone of safety as you explore the vastness of your inner world. It is strong enough to hold all that you bring into this space—every shard of grief, every ribbon of joy, every echo of the past, and every seed of future growth.

The Ritual of Ingestion: A Sacred Pact for Healing

In the realm of psychedelic-assisted psychotherapy, ingesting the medicine transcends the act of simply taking a substance—it is a ritual. This deliberate and sacred moment signifies the commencement of a profound journey. It is an act steeped in intentionality, a conscious commitment to the path of healing and self-discovery that lies ahead.

As you hold the medicine, recognize it as more than a pharmacological agent; it is a key, an instrument of transformation that will unlock doors within your psyche, some of which have perhaps been long-sealed by the scars of combat, and the burdens carried home. You stand at the threshold, and with the ingestion, you signal to yourself and your support team that you are ready to step through.

In this moment of quietude, before the medicine merges with your being, take the time to revisit and reaffirm your intentions. These intentions are the bedrock of your experience, the compass points that will guide you through the inner landscapes you're about to navigate. They are the beacons that can guide you back to a place of purpose and meaning, even when the journey grows intense or bewildering.

This ritual of ingestion is a reflective pause, a time to gather all the threads of your life—the trials and the triumphs, the pain, and the pride —and redirect them into a focused objective for the journey. Whether seeking solace, understanding, forgiveness, or growth, let each intention be clear and present as you partake in the medicine.

Engage with this act mindfully. Feel the moment's weight, the medicine's texture in your hands, and the purpose in your heart. With each breath, infuse the space with your readiness and willingness to engage with whatever arises. It is an affirmation of trust in the medicine and with the therapeutic process, your inner strength, and the people who stand sentinel to your healing.

As you ingest the medicine, you may feel a solemnity akin to a warrior's quiet before the dawn of battle. Yet, in this new kind of confrontation, your courage is turned inward, and your weapons are relinquished for the tools of introspection and openness. This ritual marks your departure from the known shores of conventional therapy into the expansive seas of the mind facilitated by psychedelics.

Allow yourself to honor the gravity of this moment and your unique journey. This is your sacred pact with healing, a profound acknowledgment of the work you are about to do. The medicine is your ally, and the intentions you set are the silent vows you make to yourself: to engage deeply, to confront fearlessly, to explore sincerely, and to emerge with new insights and clarity.

In this deliberate act of ingestion, encircled by the support of your guides and the accumulated wisdom of your own life experiences, you enact a powerful ceremony. It is a ritual that honors the past, engages the present, and reaches forth to the potential of the future. Here, you stand not at the end of a road but at a crossroads where every path forward is woven with the promise of transformation and the potential for profound healing.

Mindfulness and Presence: Breathing as an Anchor

With its roots deeply planted in ancient practices, mindfulness has found a place of honor in modern therapy for its simplicity and effectiveness. For you, the combat veteran, these techniques are not foreign; they are reminiscent of tactical breathing exercises drilled into you to maintain composure under fire. Now, these same techniques serve a different kind of battle—the inward journey through the psyche under the influence of psychedelics.

Focused breathing is your anchor. As you sit with the medicine working its way into your consciousness, the rhythm of your breath becomes a point of return, a steadying pulse amidst the uncertainty of this new terrain. Each inhalation is a reminder to return to the present moment, to ground yourself in the now, where the experience unfolds.

Just as tactical breathing has brought clarity and calm in the chaos of combat, mindfulness, and relaxation are your grounding techniques when the waves of the psychedelic experience swell and threaten to pull you under. It's not about fighting the current; rather, it's about finding your rhythm within it, allowing it to flow over and around you, to be with it without becoming overwhelmed.

Mindfulness teaches presence—being with what is, moment to moment. This presence is invaluable as you navigate the shifting land-scapes of the mind under psychedelics. It allows you to observe your thoughts and feelings without attachment and to recognize them as transient parts of your experience that come and go. This watchful state is powerful; it creates space around your experiences, allowing you to encounter and engage with them without being consumed.

Relaxation techniques—progressive muscle relaxation, guided imag-ery, or simply acknowledging and then letting go of tension in the body—can also serve as a touchstone throughout the experience. In times when the body's response might mirror the intensity of the emotional journey, these relaxation practices remind you of your ability to exert subtle control, offer yourself comfort, and maintain a center of calm within the storm.

Incorporating these practices into the experience of ingesting psy-chedelic medicine is an extension of the preparatory work you have engaged in with your therapist. It is a way to apply familiar skills to unfamiliar settings to translate the discipline and control learned in the military into the therapeutic process. Each mindful breath is a note of resilience, a beat of perseverance, and a cadence that harmonizes the internal and external.

As the journey progresses, and perhaps as your sense of time and space becomes more fluid, returning to your breath reminds you of your agency. You are not adrift in this journey; you actively engage with it, riding its ebb and flow with the assurance that your breath is a life-line—a reminder of life's continuity and enduring presence within it.

In essence, mindfulness and presence during a psychedelic session are not passive activities; they are dynamic engagements that harness your ability to stay present and composed. Just as a soldier must be aware of their surroundings, so must you be mindful of the shifting inner landscape, navigating it with the same attentiveness and steadiness. The practice of mindfulness is your tactical maneuver, the calm in the eye of the psychedelic storm, providing you with an unwavering sense of self amid the profound transformation that unfolds.

The Present Moment: Your Arena of Transformation

In the theater of combat, the critical skill of staying present can mean the difference between life and death. In the realm of psychedelic-assisted psychotherapy, the present moment holds a different kind of power—it is the arena where the battle for healing and self-discovery is fought and won. Here, you are called not to arms but to awareness.

As you embark on this journey, anchoring yourself in the now is essential. With its skirmishes and scars, the past has shaped you, and the future, with its uncertainties and possibilities, awaits you. However, neither the bygone battles nor the anticipated advances hold sway in the therapeutic space. The weight of history and the whisper of tomorrow dissolve in the present moment, leaving only the immediate experience —the unfolding reality of the here and now.

Psychedelics have a profound ability to amplify this moment, each second blooming into an eternity of sensations, emotions, and insights. This intensified sense of being can be overwhelming; however, it is within this expansive now that you find the fertile ground for change. Every breath, each heartbeat, and every nuance of thought becomes infused into the essence of your experience.

Being present is more than a passive observation; it is an active engagement with each moment as it arises. It requires a steadfast commitment to witness, without judgment, the cavalcade of inner experiences that the medicine elicits. There will be moments that beckon you back to the trenches of past trauma and others that catapult you into the realm of future anxieties. Acknowledge them, then gently guide yourself back to the present, for healing occurs only in the present.

The practice of mindfulness is your ally in this endeavor. It trains your focus, steadies your resolve, and equips you to meet each moment with equanimity. Much like life, the psychedelic journey unfolds in the present, and each second is an opportunity—an invitation—to interact with the profound truths that arise.

In this arena, there is no enemy to vanquish, no territory to seize. The present moment asks only for your full participation, courage to confront what appears, and willingness to embrace the lessons it offers. Here, the victories are not measured in conquests but in the quiet acknowledgment of pain, the acceptance of what is, and the hopeful embrace of what may yet come to be.

Embrace the present moment as your arena, where you are both the warrior and the peacemaker. In the continuous flow of now, it is here that your psychedelic journey finds its depth and meaning. Each moment is a brushstroke on the canvas of your consciousness, each a step on the path to understanding. In this space, the present moment is not just a slice of time—it is the field upon which your spirit engages in its most significant endeavor: the quest for inner peace and the return to wholeness.

The Landing: Embracing Patience and Compassion on Descent

The journey inward, under the guidance of psychedelics, can be likened to a helicopter gently descending into untamed landscapes. This is your 'Landing'—the critical transition from preparation to actualizing the experience. Just as a pilot approaches the ground with a keen awareness of conditions, you, too, must navigate this descent into your psyche with care and attention.

Patience is your first companion upon this landing. It's the understanding that healing and insight are not rushed processes. They unfold in their own time. Just as a soldier understands the importance of waiting for the right moment to act, in this inner journey, patience is what allows you to be with your experience without pushing or pulling it in any direction. Each feeling, each memory, each revelation comes at its own pace. Allow them to surface naturally, giving them the time they deserve.

Allowing is your second ally. It is the act of opening the gates of your consciousness without reservation or expectation. This is not a passive state; it's an active surrender to the journey, accepting the waves of emotions and thoughts that may arise. Allowing requires bravery—the courage to meet whatever comes your way with a steady heart.

Self-directed kindness and compassion are the nourishment needed during this landing. The realm you are entering may present challenges, and meeting them with a spirit of self-compassion is essential. Just as you would empathize with a comrade in distress, turn that gentle understanding upon yourself.

Self-love is the armor you wear into this battle. It is the shield that protects you from harsh self-judgment and the sword that cuts through the self-doubt that may arise. Embracing self-love means honoring your journey, acknowledging the effort it takes to engage in this work, and affirming your worthiness of healing and peace.

Take your time—there is no hurry. Each moment on this descent is precious and deserves your entire presence. Remember, the therapy session is a microcosm of life itself; it doesn't adhere to strict schedules or predictable patterns. As you allow the medicine to work, let your experience flow at its natural rhythm, and trust in the process.

This 'Landing' is a step in your therapeutic process and a recommitment to your journey—a journey that is unique to you. Just as a helicopter settles onto new ground with precision and grace, so too must you engage with your inner world, knowing that the wisdom it holds will reveal itself in due time. Take this descent with an open heart, and let patience, allowing, kindness, compassion, and self-love guide you to the profound understanding that awaits.

Final Thoughts Before the Leap: Embracing the Journey Within

As you approach the threshold of your psychedelic trek, it is vital to recall the essence of your military ethos—not the rigor and discipline and the profound resilience that has been instilled in you. This resilience has carried you through uncertainties and adversities that few can truly comprehend. You have navigated the landscapes of conflict and camaraderie, and now you stand at the precipice of a different kind of voyage—one that plumbs the depths of your psyche.

The leap you are about to take is unlike any before; it requires a fusion of courage and surrender. As the effects of the medicine materialize, understand that this is more than a simple process—it is a quest for wholeness and serenity. The battlefields you've known were external terrains, yet now the terrain is the vast expanse of your inner world.

In this moment, as the boundaries of the mind begin to expand, remember the strength within you. Every challenge faced, every hardship overcome, and every moment of solidarity with your brothers and sisters in arms has been a preparation for this moment of introspection and revelation.

As you relinquish control and let the journey unfold, take solace in the fortress of safety constructed by your support team. Their presence is a constant reminder that while this journey is yours alone to travel, you are enveloped by an unwavering circle of care and guardianship.

Arm yourself with an open heart and a tranquil mind, ready to encounter the myriad facets of your being. Trust in the preparation, the process, and the people who stand vigilant on your behalf. The therapeutic landscape you are about to navigate is sacred and fertile ground for growth and healing.

And so, with a breath that anchors you to the present and a spirit unbound by the past or future, step forward. Let the medicine be the key that unlocks doors within. Embrace this mission with the same bravery you have mustered in the past. This is not a surrender to the enemy but rather an embrace of the innermost self—a chance to heal, understand, and emerge transformed.

You have braved the crucible of warfare; now brace for the profound voyage of the soul. You are equipped, you are watched over, and you are ready. Welcome to the transformation of the mind—your journey to inner peace.

CHAPTER 11

The Therapeutic Psychedelic Landscape: An Overview What to Expect When You're on a Psychedelic

As combat veterans and their families consider the path of psychedelic-assisted psychotherapy, understanding what to expect during a psychedelic experience is paramount. The following sections provide a foundational understanding of the typical stages and sensations associated with the psychedelic journey, which can be profoundly personal and variable.

After ingestion, psychedelics typically take effect within 20 to 40 minutes, depending on the substance and its form. During this phase, individuals may experience a range of initial sensations, such as mild anxiety, anticipation, or changes in bodily sensations. There's often a feeling of departure from ordinary consciousness, signaling the beginning of the journey.

As the effects intensify, there's an amplification of sensory perception. Colors may become brighter, sounds more distinct, and emotional responses heightened. For many, this phase is accompanied by a sense of wonder or awe. Veterans might find themselves revisiting memories with increased vividness, which, under therapeutic guidance, can initiate the process of recontextualizing traumatic events.

The peak of a psychedelic experience can be the most intense phase. It's where the ego's hold may loosen, and one might encounter profound insights or confront challenging emotions. This period can last from a few minutes to several hours. The therapeutic setting and support are critical in helping individuals navigate turbulent emotional waters.

Following the peak, there tends to be a plateau phase where the intensity stabilizes. Veterans might be reflective during this stage, contemplating life, relationships, and self-identity. Insights gained here can be integral to the therapeutic process, fostering personal growth and healing.

As the psychedelic effects wane, individuals start to return to their baseline consciousness. This descent can be accompanied by complex and differing emotions, from relief to sadness. It's crucial to begin integrating the experience, discussing it with the therapist, and consolidating insights.

Many veterans talk about a period of 'afterglow' following the immediate experience, lasting days or weeks, where one may feel an increased sense of peace, connectedness, or well-being. It's during this phase that many report sustained therapeutic benefits, including reduced symptoms of PTSD or depression.

The journey through a psychedelic experience can be a profound and transformative process, especially when carefully guided and supported within a therapeutic context. For combat veterans, this could mean a pivotal point in healing, offering a new perspective on past experiences and a reinvigorated sense of self. Now, let us move on to what to expect with specific psychedelics. Remember, While this overview offers a general framework, individual experiences vary widely. It's also crucial to highlight that psychedelics are powerful substances, and their use should be cautiously approached within legal parameters and under professional guidance.

LSD

LSD (lysergic acid diethylamide) stands as a pillar in the study of psychedelics for therapeutic use, with a history that interweaves cultural narrative and scientific inquiry. For combat veterans embarking on this journey, LSD presents a profound opportunity for psychological transformation.

The experience typically commences within 30 to 90 minutes post-ingestion. Users may notice subtle changes as the compound takes effect—a sharpening of visual perception, a deepening of emotional understanding, or a gentle shift in their thought patterns. This phase often carries a sense of anticipation akin to the moments before dawn.

As the experience deepens, a sensory performance begins. Visuals may include geometric patterns, intensified colors, or tracers. Auditory senses are heightened, with sounds acquiring new textures and dimensions. This sensory augmentation is not merely an alteration but an expansion, offering a broader palette with which one perceives the world.

Emotionally, LSD can evoke a spectrum of feelings, from euphoria to introspection. Veterans may find emotional barriers becoming permeable, allowing access to a wellspring of previously guarded memories and feelings. Cognitively, thoughts can become less linear, less constrained by habitual patterns, fostering novel insights or reevaluating past experiences.

The peak of an LSD experience is often where the most significant therapeutic potential lies. This period is marked by an intense introspective state that can last several hours. Here, many report a sense of unity with the universe, ego dissolution, or profound realizations about their life's narrative. The therapeutic setting provides a vital anchor, ensuring these insights are framed within a healing context.

The gradual return to baseline consciousness is accompanied by a period of integration. For veterans, this is a time to reflect on the journey with the aid of their therapist. The recontextualization of trauma may have begun, and the insights gleaned now need to be integrated into daily lives. This process is not immediate but unfolds over days to weeks as the experience is assimilated.

Post-experience, individuals may enter a state of 'afterglow,' where the insights and emotional shifts linger. This period is often characterized by a sense of calm, decreased anxiety, and a more optimistic outlook. For combat veterans, this can translate to a respite from the persistent shadow of PTSD and an opening toward continued healing and growth.

It is imperative to underscore the importance of set and setting, especially for individuals with a history of trauma. A supportive, controlled environment and guidance from a trained professional are essential to navigate the powerful effects of LSD safely.

LSD offers a canvas for the psyche, where veterans can explore the contours of their inner landscape with fresh eyes. Its therapeutic potential is rooted in its ability to foster a profound

level of introspection and emotional release, set within a structure that honors the complexity of the human experience. As research evolves, so does our understanding of how to harness these experiences for healing and transformation.

Note: The use of LSD, like any psychedelic substance, should be undertaken with caution and always within the boundaries of the law and under the supervision of qualified medical and mental health professionals. The information provided here is for educational purposes and should not be considered an endorsement or recommendation for unsupervised use.

Psilocybin

Psilocybin is the psychoactive compound found in 'magic mushrooms.' It has gained recognition for its potential to relieve psychological distress. In the landscape of psychedelic-assisted therapy, psilocybin offers a unique journey into the self, one that can be especially poignant for veterans grappling with the aftermath of combat and the associated psychological scars.

The psilocybin journey often commences with a feeling of warmth and emotional softening. As the compound starts to take effect, which can be anywhere from 20 to 40 minutes after ingestion, individuals may experience a wave of relaxation and dissolution of internal resistance, setting the stage for deeper introspection.

Gradually, as the psilocybin experience intensifies, there is an escalation in emotional and sensory engagement. Users often report an enhanced sense of connection to their surroundings, empathy, and a profound sense of interconnectedness. These sensations are coupled with vivid visual enhancements, where colors and textures may appear more profound and mesmerizing.

For veterans, the psilocybin experience can become a navigational tool for the psyche, steering through layers of consciousness and revealing insights. This can manifest as revisiting memories with a new perspective, often leading to a reframing or re-interpretation of past events, which is a crucial step in the therapeutic process for conditions like PTSD.

The peak of a psilocybin experience is marked by the potential for cathartic emotional release. Many individuals confront and work through their deepest traumas in this transformative phase. It's a time when the sense of self may dissolve, often referred to as 'ego-death,' which can be both unsettling and liberating, paving the way for a renewed sense of self.

As the intensity of the peak subsides, individuals enter a reflective phase. This is an essential period for integration, where the revelations and emotional shifts experienced can be processed and understood. Veterans and their therapists can start contextualizing their insights, making sense of them in relation to their past experiences and current life situations.

Following the session, an 'afterglow' effect may persist, where individuals experience prolonged benefits. These can include enhanced mood, a sense of peace, and decreased symptoms of depression and anxiety. The clarity gained from the psilocybin experience can be instrumental in providing veterans with a new outlook on life, promoting lasting psychological growth.

It is crucial to approach psilocybin sessions with mindfulness and under the guidance of a trained professional, especially for individuals with complex trauma histories. Set and setting, alongside therapeutic support, are vital to ensure a safe and healing experience.

Psilocybin offers a unique therapeutic journey, one that has the potential to act as an inner healer, especially for veterans facing the challenges of PTSD and related conditions. It provides a pathway for exploring the psyche, promoting healing, and facilitating a profound reconnection with oneself and the world. As with all psychedelic substances, psilocybin should be approached with respect, in a controlled environment, and with professional support to navigate its powerful effects.

Note: It's essential for those interested in psilocybin-assisted therapy to consult with healthcare professionals and to consider the legal status of the substance in their region. The experiences and outcomes can vary significantly from person to person, and the information provided here does not substitute for professional medical advice.

DMT

DMT (Dimethyltryptamine) is often referred to as the 'spirit molecule.' It is a naturally occurring psychedelic that is also the active ingredient in ayahuasca, a traditional Amazonian brew. It is known for its rapid onset and intensely vivid psychedelic experience.

When ingested, especially as part of an ayahuasca ceremony, DMT induces a powerful altered state of consciousness that typically lasts between 2 to 6 hours. The experience is often described as a journey or voyage characterized by complex visions, deep emotional revelations, and a sense of traversing various planes of existence.

Combat veterans may find that DMT facilitates an intense confrontation with past traumas, sometimes personified in visual or narrative forms, allowing for a therapeutic reprocessing of these experiences in a ceremonial and structured setting. This can significantly reduce stress and professional burnout symptoms and provide a scaffold for mental health improvements.

5-MeO-DMT, often dubbed the 'God molecule,' is another naturally occurring psychedelic compound, which, despite being similar in structure to DMT, offers a notably different experience. Derived from the venom of the Bufo Alvarius toad or synthesized in a lab, it is known for its rapid and intense effects.

5-MeO-DMT's effects are often felt within seconds of inhalation and can last anywhere from 30 minutes to an hour. Unlike DMT's colorful and narrative-rich experience, 5-MeO-DMT is characterized by a nondual, often described as a unitive experience, where individuals report encountering a boundless, formless state of being or consciousness.

For veterans, this can mean a temporary dissolution of the self or ego, which can be both disorienting and enlightening. In therapeutic settings, this brief but profound journey can allow individuals to step beyond their personal narratives and traumas, potentially leading to re-evaluating their life experiences and sense of identity.

The principal difference between DMT and 5-MeO-DMT lies in the nature of the experiences they induce. DMT is known for its narrative, often highly visual journey that can connect users with various emotions and 'otherworldly' encounters. 5-MeO-DMT, in contrast, is less about visual storytelling and more about a profound sense of oneness and existential insight, with less emphasis on the visual component and more on the sensation of merging with a greater consciousness.

Given their potency and the depth of the altered states, they induce, both DMT and 5-MeO-DMT should be approached with the utmost respect and caution. Combat veterans considering these substances for therapeutic purposes should do so only under the supervision of professionals trained in psychedelic-assisted therapy and within a legal framework.

DMT and 5-MeO-DMT offer profound, albeit different, psychological exploration and healing pathways. For combat veterans, the intense and often rapid experiences provided by these substances can lead to significant therapeutic outcomes, especially when appropriately integrated within a structured and supportive setting.

Note: The use of DMT and 5-MeO-DMT for therapeutic purposes is a complex subject that requires careful consideration of legal, medical, and psychological factors. It is imperative to engage with these substances within the context of professional guidance and to respect the boundaries of legality and safety.

MDMA

MDMA, a substance historically associated with social and recreational use, has been reconceptualized in recent years as a potential linchpin in the treatment of PTSD. Clinical research has illustrated that MDMA can significantly enhance the process of fear extinction and aid in the reconsolidation of traumatic memories, providing a beacon of hope for those who have found little relief from conventional treatment modalities (Feduccia et al., 2018).

The concept of a "therapeutic window" is critical when understanding the role of MDMA in treatment settings. This window refers to the optimal psychological state induced by MDMA, characterized by a remarkable decrease in the defensive emotional responses usually triggered by recalling traumatic events. In this state, veterans may find themselves able to explore and process painful memories with a level of emotional engagement that was previously inaccessible to them.

MDMA induces a unique state of introspection, wherein individuals report a heightened sense of clarity and connection to their emotions. This state is marked by a reduction in self-criticism and an increase in self-compassion, which can be particularly beneficial for veterans who may struggle with self-blame and guilt in relation to their combat experiences.

Physiologically, MDMA users may experience a range of sensations, such as a warming of the body, a feeling of lightness, and a gentle stimulation that contrasts with the jitteriness associated with other stimulants. While these sensations can enhance the therapeutic experience, it is the emotional and cognitive shifts that are of primary interest in the context of PTSD treatment.

Post-session integration is a cornerstone of the therapeutic process. The insights and shifts experienced during the MDMA session are not autonomous; they require careful and continued psychological work to be fully integrated into the individual's life and to effect lasting change.

Despite its potential, MDMA is not without risks. Side effects can include, but are not limited to, dehydration, nausea, and, on rarer occasions, more serious adverse effects. Thus, the therapeutic use of MDMA must always be supervised by medical and psychological professionals to ensure safety and efficacy.

The potential of MDMA in facilitating emotional processing and engagement in the context of PTSD represents a significant development in psychotherapy. For veterans facing the often insurmountable challenges of PTSD, MDMA-assisted therapy could serve as a vital tool in their healing journey, offering a renewed connection to life beyond the shadow of trauma.

Note: It is crucial to highlight that MDMA-assisted therapy is currently limited to clinical research settings and should only be undertaken with licensed professionals in a controlled environment.

Mescaline

Mescaline: As we venture further into the realms of psychedelic-assisted psychotherapy, mescaline stands out as a substance with a long history of sacramental use, particularly among Native American cultures. Its potential for psychotherapeutic use is emerging, as anecdotal and early clinical evidence point to its capacity for catalyzing deep psychological insight and an expansive sense of connectedness.

Mescaline, a phenethylamine primarily derived from the Peyote cactus, induces a state often characterized by a profound sense of interconnectedness with the world. The experience can be vibrant visual enhancements, emotional intensification, and philosophical contemplation. Users commonly report increased sensitivity to aesthetic elements of their environment, such as colors, patterns, and sounds, which can take on a new significance and depth.

The mescaline experience often entails an amplification of sensory perception. Visual effects may include geometric patterns and intensified colors, while auditory sensations can seem richer and more nuanced. This heightened sensory input can lead to a renewed appreciation of nature, art, and music, often described as re-encountering the world with a fresh sense of wonder.

Psychologically, mescaline can foster a significant degree of introspection, facilitating access to emotionally charged memories and re-evaluating personal beliefs and life choices. When guided by a therapist, this reflective state can help veterans recontextualize past experiences and foster personal growth.

Many mescaline users describe spiritual experiences, including feelings of unity with a greater consciousness of the universe. This aspect of the mescaline experience can lead to profound existential reflections and a re-examination of one's place within the larger web of life, which can be therapeutic, especially for individuals feeling disconnected or isolated.

As with all psychedelics, the experience of mescaline is deeply influenced by set and setting. Preparing for a session with a clear intention in a safe and supportive environment can significantly impact the quality and outcomes of the experience.

While contemporary research is still in the early stages, the therapeutic potential of mescaline for veterans is supported by its historical use for healing and spiritual exploration. It is believed to assist individuals in accessing and processing complex emotional material in a profound and transformative manner.

The safety profile of mescaline, particularly in a controlled therapeutic context, remains under investigation. Common side effects may include nausea and increased heart rate, emphasizing the need for medical oversight during use.

The traditional use of mescaline as a tool for insight and connection offers a promising avenue for therapeutic exploration. As a 'teacher of the desert,' it may provide combat veterans a pathway to profound personal and spiritual growth, alongside the potential for psychological healing.

Note: It's important to note that mescaline is classified as a Schedule I controlled substance in the United States, and its use outside of sanctioned religious ceremonies or approved research settings is illegal.

Ketamine

Ketamine: Within the context of psychedelic-assisted psychotherapy, ketamine occupies a unique niche. Unlike classic psychedelics, its primary action is as a dissociative anesthetic. Still, at sub-anesthetic doses, it exhibits rapid-acting antidepressant effects. This has profound implications for its use in therapeutic settings, particularly for combat veterans grappling with persistent and intrusive traumatic memories.

When ingested at these lower doses, ketamine can induce a state that is often described as dissociative, which means that it can create a sense of detachment from one's immediate reality, including a temporary disconnection from physical and emotional pain. This experience can create a therapeutic window of opportunity for patients to explore difficult memories or thoughts with less emotional intensity.

The dissociative state induced by ketamine is one where patients often report feeling separated from their body or sense of self. This can manifest as a feeling of floating, flying, or even journeying through different environments. This altered state of consciousness can help interrupt entrenched patterns of negative thinking or rumination, often associated with depression and PTSD.

Ketamine's most striking feature in the realm of mental health is its ability to produce rapid antidepressant effects. This phenomenon has garnered significant interest from the medical community. Studies suggest that ketamine may promote synaptogenesis, the formation of new synapses, which could potentially reverse the synaptic deficits caused by chronic stress and depression (Krystal et al., 2019).

Veterans who have experienced ketamine therapy often report a sense of cognitive flexibility following their sessions. This state can allow for new perspectives and insights into old wounds, providing an invaluable space for therapeutic work. The dissociative effect offers a respite from the constant barrage of traumatic memories, giving room for reflection and the reorganization of thought processes.

While the dissociative effects of ketamine can be therapeutic, they can also be disorienting. A well-structured therapeutic environment with trained professionals can help guide the individual through the experience, ensuring safety and maximizing the therapeutic benefits.

Ketamine is generally well-tolerated in a clinical setting, with transient side effects such as dizziness, nausea, or increased blood pressure. However, it's essential to consider the potential for dissociation to become distressing without proper support, highlighting the importance of a controlled setting and professional guidance.

Ketamine's role as a 'dissociative bridge' in the treatment of PTSD and depression represents a significant advancement in psychedelic-assisted psychotherapy. For combat veterans, it offers a reprieve from psychological distress and the possibility of gaining new, healing perspectives on traumatic experiences. With its rapid-acting nature, ketamine stands as a promising agent in the ongoing quest for effective mental health treatments.

Note: Remember that the use of ketamine for psychotherapeutic purposes should only occur under the supervision of qualified professionals within the bounds of clinical protocols.

Ibogaine

Ibogaine is a naturally occurring psychoactive substance found in plants in the Apocynaceae family. Unlike other psychedelics, ibogaine is often lauded for its potential in addiction treatment, particularly with substances such as opioids, stimulants, and alcohol. Its use in psycho-therapy, especially for combat veterans, is of interest due to its unique psychological and physiological effects.

The experience of ingesting ibogaine is often described as a profound journey that can last for up to 24-36 hours. During this time, individ-uals might undergo an intense reflective process where they revisit past experiences, including traumas or significant events. Ibogaine's effects can be divided into several phases:

> **Acute Phase:** This initial phase is characterized by visions and a dream-like state. Users often report complex, vivid imagery and a narrative that unfolds, revealing aspects of their subconscious mind.

> **Evaluative Phase:** Following the acute phase, individuals gener-ally enter a period of introspection, evaluating their life choices and experiences. This can be particularly poignant for combat veterans, as they may confront memories and emotions related to their service.

> **Resolution Phase:** In the final phase, the individual may feel a sense of resolution or acceptance. This can lead to insights inte-gral to the therapeutic process, offering a fresh perspective and potential reintegration of traumatic events with a new under-standing.

The therapeutic potential of ibogaine lies in its ability to facilitate deep psychological exploration and its reported ability to interrupt the process of addictive behavior. This interruption can provide a 'reset' for individuals suffering from substance use disorders, which is often a comorbid condition in veterans with PTSD.

Ibogaine also has significant physiological effects. It has been shown to modulate neurotransmission, affecting serotonin and opioid systems, which may explain its potential in reducing withdrawal symptoms and cravings (Brown & Alper, 2017).

It is essential to note that ibogaine is not without risks. It can have serious cardiovascular side effects, including the potential to prolong the QT interval, which can lead to life-threatening heart arrhythmias. Therefore, medical supervision in a clinical setting is critical when undergoing an ibogaine experience.

For combat veterans, ibogaine presents an opportunity for a profound inner journey that can be therapeutic, especially within the framework of psychedelic-assisted psychotherapy. It requires careful consideration, preparation, and professional guidance to ensure safety and maximize potential benefits. While it is not a panacea, ibogaine's unique properties make it an important substance to consider in the treatment of complex conditions like PTSD and addiction.

Note: Due to the significant risks associated with ibogaine, its use should be considered only under strict medical supervision and not be undertaken lightly.

As we conclude this chapter, we have established a foundational understanding of various psychedelics, each with its own unique profile and potential to catalyze psychological healing. The journey through the landscape of these powerful substances illuminates their capacity to unlock new pathways of thought, emotion, and perception, particularly for those who have endured the hardships of combat.

The substances we have examined—LSD, psilocybin, MDMA, DMT, 5-MeO-DMT, mescaline, ketamine, and ibogaine—share the common potential to offer therapeutic benefits. Yet, they differ significantly in their effects, duration, and suitability for individuals with different needs. From the unity and connectedness facilitated by LSD to the introspective depth prompted by psilocybin and the empathogenic qualities of MDMA, each psychedelic presents a different avenue for exploration and healing.

It is paramount that such potent tools are approached with caution, respect, and a clear understanding of their power. This means adhering to structured, clinically supervised settings where safety protocols are rigorously followed, and the psychological groundwork can be properly laid for the experiences these substances facilitate.

The psychotherapeutic use of psychedelics is not about casual experimentation; it is about creating a controlled environment where one can harness the profound effects of these substances to foster deep healing and personal growth. The invisible scars of combat—manifest as PTSD, moral injury, or substance use disorders—require careful, professional attention, and psychedelics, under the right conditions, may provide a path to recovery that was previously obscured.

As we transition from the direct experiences invoked by psychedelics to the critical period that follows, we must underscore the significance of integration. The insights and breakthroughs that arise during psychedelic experiences can be fleeting if not anchored adequately through reflective practices and therapeutic guidance. The next chapter will delve into the aftermath: integrating the often intense and revelatory psychedelic experiences into daily life, ensuring that the lessons learned and the growth attained have a lasting, transformative impact.

Remember, the journey does not end when the effects of the psychedelic fade; indeed, the true work may just be beginning. Integration is the key to translating extraordinary states into enduring traits, turning ephemeral moments of clarity into sustained enlightenment and well-being.

Note to the Reader: This guide underscores the essential nature of professional help in the context of psychedelic-assisted psychotherapy. While the therapeutic potential of psychedelics is substantial, they must be navigated with the utmost care, ethical consideration, and scientific rigor. Combat veterans and their families seeking this form of therapy should do so only with accredited professionals in a legally sanctioned context.

PART IV

Post Psychedelic
Therapy

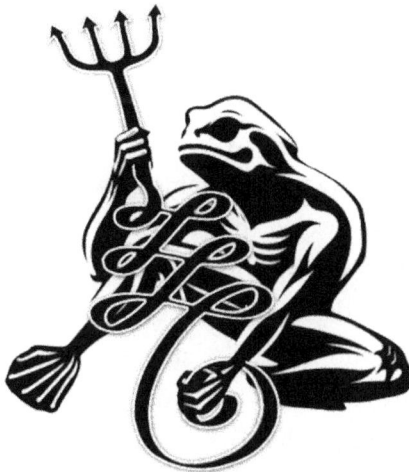

CHAPTER 12

The Return Home–
Embracing the Unfolding

Navigating the Return to *Normalcy*

For combat veterans emerging from psychedelic therapy, the notion of 'normalcy' becomes interwoven with new threads of consciousness. The conclusion of a psychedelic journey is not an end but a rite of passage into a richer psychological terrain. These brave souls, having traversed the kaleidoscopic landscapes of their minds, stand on the precipice of what many would call the 'real world.' Yet, their eyes have been opened to realities that are anything but ordinary.

In this delicate juncture, the term 'integration' becomes the veteran's mantra, but it is a task easier said than done. The profound insights and altered perceptions from the psychedelic depths demand a reconstruction of daily life. Normalcy, as it was once understood, has been irrevocably altered. Veterans find themselves equipped with a new psychological lexicon. The world they return to speaks an archaic dialect, unversed in the nuances of their expanded consciousness.

This process can be disorienting, as integrating such experiences into the veteran's psyche and life is not akin to a hero's return in classical epics—no triumphal procession or laurel wreath is awaiting. Instead, there's a subtle realization that the journey never truly ends. Each day becomes a microcosm of their psychedelic experience, with its own set of trials and revelations.

In this light, the return to 'normalcy' is a misleading term. It suggests glancing backward to a state of being that no longer fits the expanded self. Combat veterans face the formidable task of not merely returning but redefining their existence in a world that has remained static while they have transformed.

This redefinition requires recalibrating one's sense of self and the external world. Veterans must navigate through their relationships, careers, and self-care routines while integrating the profound lessons from their journeys. It's akin to trying to fit the vast ocean of their experiences into the narrow riverbeds of societal norms and expectations. It is not enough to simply step back into old routines and patterns; these individuals are called to craft a new 'normal,' one that acknowledges the breadth and depth of their psychedelic insights.

In this transformative aftermath, a potent, if not provocative, question exists: Can society make room for these transformed individuals, or is it the individual's responsibility to carve out a space within society? This new chapter in their lives challenges the veterans and the communities they return to. It asks for understanding and space for an evolutionary process that has the power to reshape individuals and perhaps society itself.

The journey back to 'normalcy' is, therefore, a misnomer. What unfolds is an emergence into a state of being that honors the wisdom gained from the psychedelic experience and seeks to infuse everyday life with this expanded awareness. It is a path that beckons the veteran to become a pioneer and live in a world that is only beginning to understand the potential of such transcendent experiences.

This chapter sets forth on this path, exploring the challenges of reintegration and the profound opportunities for personal and societal transformation that await those who dare to venture into the unknown territories of the mind.

Reintegration Challenges: Navigating Emotional Rapid

As veterans resurface from the profound depths of psychedelic therapy, they are often met with a psychological landscape that is at once richly familiar yet disconcertingly altered. The reintegration into their former lives is not a seamless transition but a journey through emotional rapids, each twist and turn demanding a fortitude akin to that of their combat experiences, yet of a vastly different nature.

The emotional upheaval that follows is not merely a series of waves to be weathered but a tidal force that reshapes the shoreline of the psyche. Psychedelic experiences have the uncanny ability to dredge up the sediment of long-suppressed emotions, laying bare the raw materials of the soul in vivid relief. Once veiled by stoic facades necessary in combat, these emotions must be confronted and reconciled.

Veterans may find themselves grappling with an emotional spectrum that is as broad as it is intense. They might encounter a newfound sensitivity to the emotional currents flowing through their daily interactions, an unsettling vulnerability where there was once impenetrable armor and an emotional acuity that cuts through the facades of everyday life. This can leave them feeling exposed in a world that seems to operate at a superficial depth.

The social navigation required in this post-psychedelic landscape can be daunting. Attempts to communicate the transformative inner journey to those who have not shared this experience can feel like speaking a foreign dialect in one's native country. No matter how well-intentioned, friends and family may struggle to bridge the gap between their understanding and the veteran's lived reality. This dissonance can amplify the veteran's sense of isolation, underscoring the need for a compassionate and patient communal response.

Indeed, it is within social interactions that many veterans feel the full weight of their journey. The challenge lies in translating the ineffable lessons and insights of their psychedelic experiences into everyday life—a currency that often seems devalued by comparison to the richness of understanding they now possess.

The reintegration process, therefore, is not merely about finding one's footing on familiar terrain. It is about learning to walk anew, with a different sense of balance and purpose. The veterans' external world may not have changed, but their internal compass has been recalibrated, often pointing to a horizon that others cannot yet see.

To navigate these emotional rapids, veterans require the lifejackets of support and understanding from their communities and the oars of personal agency to steer through the tumultuous waters. It is a process that asks them to become cartographers of their emotional landscapes, mapping out a course that honors their past experiences and present transformations.

Society has a provocative question: Are we ready to expand our collective emotional bandwidth to welcome home the profoundly changed souls of these veterans? Are we prepared to construct bridges of empathy and communication strong enough to bear the weight of their transformed selves?

This section of the chapter dares to delve deep into the inner sanctums that await veterans post-psychedelic therapy, exploring the richness of their emotional resurgence, the complexities of their social re-engagement, and the potential for both personal and communal growth. It is a call to arms for a different kind of bravery—the courage to face one's inner world with the same steadfastness as facing the battlefield.

Identity Transformation: The Alchemy of Self-Perception

The journey into the self that psychedelics precipitate is no less than alchemical. It is a process that promises not the transmutation of base metals into gold but the transformation of the psyche from a state of confinement to boundless possibility. For the combat veteran, this metamorphosis is a profound re-envisioning of identity that transcends the superficiality of change—a deep, cellular reorganization of self-perception.

This alchemy of identity is marked not by subtle shifts but by tectonic realignments of the veteran's internal landscape. The veteran, who has known a life of disciplined structure and sharply defined roles, finds themselves in the throes of a psychological maelstrom where the very pillars of their self-conception are shaken and even uprooted. The transformation is radical—a deconstruction of old belief systems, a disintegration of the ego as it was once known, and a genesis of openness to entirely new paradigms of thought.

As the veteran emerges from the chrysalis of their psychedelic experience, they often carry with them an embryonic sense of purpose. This nascent purpose, however, is not a return to the familiar comfort of old narratives but a courageous step into a reimagined existence. The identities they once held dear, often woven into the fabric of their being through military life, begin to unravel, revealing the contours of a more expansive self.

This process of self-evolution, while liberating, is not without its disquieting moments. The dissolution of long-held self-narratives can feel like a betrayal of one's past, a stepping away from the camaraderie and shared experiences that defined the veteran's sense of reality. It can be akin to a linguistic shift where the veteran must learn to speak a new dialect of self, richer and more nuanced but initially unfamiliar and daunting.

For the combat veteran, the shift can be especially striking. The ethos of military life, with its emphasis on discipline, hierarchy, and collective identity, contrasts sharply with the fluidity and individualism that often result from psychedelic therapy. It is a journey from the constricting armor of a defined persona to the unbounded realm of a fluid identity, where the concept of self is open to interpretation and reinvention.

As they stand at this crossroads of identity, veterans face a provocative charge: to navigate the reconstruction of their self-perception without a template, drawing instead from the wellspring of their inner experiences. It is a creative act, a bricolage of past experiences and newfound insights, forged into an identity containing multitudes—the warrior, the healer, the sage, and the seeker.

This chapter, therefore, delves into the heart of what it means to transform one's identity in the aftermath of psychedelic therapy. It explores the profound ways in which the self is altered and reborn. It invites the reader to witness the unfolding of this transformation, understand the gravity of such a shift, and contemplate the boundless potential that such an evolution holds for the individual veteran and the very nature of identity itself.

Anecdote: My Journey of Self-Reinvention

I have worn the emblem of a Navy SEAL—a paragon of discipline and mental fortitude—yet this was merely a minute chapter in the epic of my life. I carry the invisible scars from my time before and during military service, and my transition to civilian life was a daunting journey across a treacherous internal landscape. I battled with angst, anger, and a lingering sense of displacement. The rigid structure I knew as a warrior seemed out of sync with the fluidity required in civilian life. Even with my immersion into the depths of Buddhist and transpersonal psychology and my ascent through the demanding realms of clinical education, there was still an undercurrent of restlessness, a silent murmur of discord within me.

I wrestled with this dichotomy for decades—on the outside composed, yet there churned persistent turbulence beneath the surface. My arsenal included years of contemplative practice, psychological insights, and clinical expertise, but the undercurrent remained.

My serendipitous encounter with psychedelic-assisted psychotherapy marked the beginning of a significant transformation. Post-psychedelic therapy, I found liberation from the tumultuous emotions that had long entangled me. The anger and frustration that I had carried dissipated, revealing them to be shadows rather than shackles, and in their absence, I discovered a serenity that was new to me. This awakening wasn't a physical rebirth but a revitalization of spirit and purpose. Where once there was inner turmoil, now there was calm; where there had been exhaustion, there was relentless energy.

But this profound shift brought its own set of challenges. Just as reintegration into civilian life posed difficulties after military service, reintegration after psychedelic therapy presented its unique hurdles. The changes were profound, reshaping my identity, worldview, and even how I perceived my own life—a life that perhaps had been constructed through a lens of discord.

Once the veil was lifted, I realized that what I had built might no longer serve me. These challenges were daunting, yet they sprouted from a place of peace and consciousness I hadn't known before, making them more aligned with my authentic self, less discordant, and more harmonious.

This transformation touched every aspect of my existence. My relationships, career, spirituality, and—most critically—my relationship with myself evolved. The once rigid confines that overshadowed my life morphed into a profound appreciation for compassion, unity, diversity, and collaborative spirit. The warrior mindset I held for so long didn't disappear; instead, it merged with my present self, forming a distinctive blend of resilience and empathy.

My journey through psychedelic therapy was a venture into deep self-reflection, transcending what conventional therapy could reach. It was like threading through the eye of a needle, emerging into the expanse of my consciousness, now open and ready to be navigated. This inner exploration wasn't a solo quest; it was supported by professionals who expertly balanced the psyche's potential for transformation with the necessity for grounded integration.

My story is unique to me yet reflects the experiences of many veterans on a similar path. The narrative offers a perspective on the veteran's return—not as a solitary retreat from combat but as ongoing discovery and renewal.

The Continuum of Metamorphosis

The threshold that marks the end of a psychedelic experience heralds not a conclusion but the commencement of a profound continuum of metamorphosis. For the combat veteran, this transition is a sacred pilgrimage from the battlefields to the inner sanctums of the psyche—a journey laden with revelations, resilience, and renewal. Within this continuum of metamorphoses, the raw materials of past experiences are alchemized, forging a renewed sense of self.

As veterans go through this complex process, they engage in a careful interaction with a constantly evolving reality. The fabric of their psyche, previously shaped by the lasting effects of combat, now incorporates new patterns of thought and emotion. They become explorers of their inner worlds, mapping out challenging and exhilarating areas. Reintegration will not be easy; it is complex, often convoluted, and punctuated with breakthroughs and setbacks. It is a domain where the conventional metrics of progress are rendered obsolete, supplanted by the profound realization that healing is not linear but cyclical—spiral in nature, echoing the ancient wisdom of countless traditions.

Families and communities, standing as witnesses and allies to this transformative process, play an instrumental role. The foundation of support they build is vital to the veteran's journey. It is a synergy of patience, education, and the sacred act of holding space for the unfurling of a new chapter in a veteran's life.

This book has endeavored to journey alongside you, offering a compass to navigate the terrain beyond the psychedelic experience. The narratives, insights, and perspectives presented herein are not merely academic or philosophical musings—they are lifelines cast into the waters of change, meant to steady you as you traverse your unique passage.

The true north of this journey is not a return to who we were but an awakening to who we can become. It is about embracing the perpetual evolution of our being, recognizing that each moment offers a chance for rebirth. As we close this chapter, let it be known that the journey does not end here—it merely takes a new direction, guided by the stars of introspection, growth, and the unyielding courage that defines the heart of a warrior.

For every veteran emerging from the psychedelic experience, remember you are not merely returning to life; you are redefining it. Carry forth the wisdom gleaned from your inner and outer journeys, and step boldly into the unfolding narrative of your existence. This is your quest, a path marked by the footprints of giants and the whispers of ancestors, leading you not back to where you began but forward to where you belong.

CHAPTER 13

The Psychedelic Reawakening – Healing the Invisible Wounds

As combat veterans emerge from the profound depths of psychedelic therapy, many report a transformative spiritual awakening. This seismic shift in consciousness is marked by an acute realization of the interwoven nature of existence. The spiritual self, previously shrouded by the fog of everyday reality, begins to unveil itself, initiating a journey of existential discovery that defies the ordinary.

Veterans recount voyages that pierce through the veil of mundane perception, leading to a space where their spiritual identity is illuminated. It is within this inner cosmos, often obscured in the day-to-day, that they encounter enduring truths. While eternal and omnipresent, these truths had eluded their grasp until these profound moments of clarity.

Interconnectedness, a cornerstone of the psychedelic experience, brings a dissolution of ego and a recognition of life's intricacies. Veterans find themselves integral parts, individual yet inseparable from the majestic whole. Here, the notion of spiritual resilience is birthed, paralleling the rebirth of the mythical phoenix. They understand life's impermanence and unity with the cosmos from the ashes of their traumatic past.

Navigating the existential currents with newfound purpose, veterans discover within themselves the archetype of the spiritual warrior. This warrior wields not weapons but the virtues of empathy, insight, and a profound grasp of the ephemeral nature of suffering. Their battles are no longer against external foes but against the shadows within, seeking a peace that is both internal and universal.

Integrating these psychedelic insights catalyzes a transformation in the veteran's identity. As the old self-concept dissolves, they begin to construct a fresh understanding that honors their past while embracing the endless possibilities of the future. Life, death, and one's role in the grander scheme take on new meaning, continuously evolving with each revelation imparted by the psychedelic journey.

Within this transformative process, veterans recognize that the microcosm of their being mirrors the vast macrocosm of the universe. A sense of sacred awe and respect for the cosmic dance ensues as they acknowledge the universe's presence around them and its resonance within. This expanded cosmic consciousness bestows upon them the serene power to act with deep empathy and unity, allowing them to partake in the unfolding story of existence with a tranquil fortitude.

The passage through spiritual and existential awakening that psychedelics facilitate can be profoundly healing for veterans. This metamorphosis provides a new framework through which they can understand their experiences and a navigational tool for traversing internal storms. The resultant spiritual resilience and existential grounding can offer solace to the soul and fuel a fervent engagement with the full spectrum of life approached with balanced wonder and bravery.

The Blossoming of Emotional Resilience

The journey through and beyond the gauntlet of military service, particularly combat, can leave an indelible mark on the psyche. Traditional therapies for veterans with PTSD and related conditions often focus on building a form of resilience—a kind of emotional armor to shield them from life's adversities. However, what unfolds post-psychedelic experience is reported to be different. It is a blossoming of a softer, more permeable form of resilience that does not repel emotional distress but moves with and through it, allowing a person to experience the full spectrum of human emotions without being capsized by them. The fabric of self-compassion, often frayed by the self-critical narratives internalized during and after combat, begins to be rewoven in the aftermath of psychedelic experiences. Veterans recount moments of profound self-forgiveness—times when they could finally separate their sense of self from their actions or the actions they witnessed. This self-compassion allows them to move forward with a gentler, more forgiving inner dialogue, which becomes a cornerstone for enduring resilience.

The static and often stormy emotional landscape veterans navigate can transform into a dynamic terrain where emotions are neither suppressed nor overwhelming. They recount tales of recognizing their emotional triggers yet feeling a sense of control and understanding that they had not experienced before. The landscape no longer feels like a minefield but rather like varied topography, navigable and rich with life's authentic expressions.

The stories from veterans are powerful. They speak to the potential of psychedelics to fortify emotional resilience. These narratives are not mere anecdotes; they are lived experiences that underscore the shift from surviving to thriving. Whether returning to a long-abandoned hobby with joy or facing a challenging relationship with renewed hope, these tales paint a picture of life's transformation through the lens of increased emotional resilience.

This newfound resilience is not an isolated phenomenon but echoes through veteran communities. Support groups and therapy sessions are replete with stories of change and adaptation, resonating with others and often instilling a sense of possibility and hope. The resonance within these communities doesn't just reinforce individual resilience; it creates a contagion of strength, supporting a network of healing that includes family, friends, and fellow veterans.

The post-psychedelic experience is a bridge between the isolation of emotional distress and the mainland of shared human experience. In this bridged space, emotional resilience finds its true expression as a personal triumph and a collective gain. This resilience is a beacon for combat veterans, guiding them back to themselves and the relationships that enrich their lives. The shared human experience, once dimmed by the shadow of trauma, begins to shine through the interactions with loved ones, the community, and, most importantly, the self.

As veterans continue their journey beyond the psychedelic experience, the seeds of resilience that have been planted require nurturing. Therapeutic work, ongoing self-care practices, and community support are the sunlight, water, and soil that ensure these seeds grow into strong, lasting attributes. This cultivation is not always linear or straightforward. It is a path marked by hope and the potential for a full and emotionally resilient life.

The psychedelic reawakening offers a vista of emotional resilience characterized not by an impenetrable shield but by a flexible willow that bends with the winds of emotional turmoil and remains rooted. The accounts of those who have walked this path illuminate a way forward for others, marking a journey from the confines of trauma to the expansive realm of emotional strength and flexibility.

Cognitive Flexibility: The Mind's Agile Dance

Within the chrysalis of the psychedelic experience, there is an opportunity for profound cognitive metamorphosis. This transformation, akin to the mind's agile dance, represents a departure from the calcified patterns forged in the heat of combat and the chilling aftermath of reintegration struggles. Psychedelics have been reported to serve as a catalyst for this cognitive renaissance, softening the rigid molds of past beliefs and springing forth flexibility of both thought and action.

Psychedelics can act as a solvent, dissolving the adhesive that binds veterans to outworn paradigms. This mental pivot is not merely a release from the old but an embrace of the new—an adoption of thought patterns that are innovative and adaptive. Within the context of psychedelic-assisted psychotherapy, the crystallized narratives of self and world can melt into a fluid mosaic of possibilities, affording the individual a broadened perspective that is ripe for growth.

The stories from the hearts and minds of those who have served are rich with examples of newfound plasticity in problem-solving and creativity. The utility of this flexibility is tangible, from the veteran who approaches interpersonal conflicts with newfound diplomacy to the one who discovers unexpected solutions to logistical hurdles in their civilian job. This enhanced cognitive flexibility can manifest as a reinvigorated ability to imagine, create, and innovate.

In the reframing of reality, psychedelics offer a lens through which the world is not only seen but also interpreted anew. This section will delve into the poignant moments when long-held, unchallengeable beliefs are revisited and reshaped under the influence of these substances. With the integration of psychedelic experiences, veterans find that they can reconstruct their understanding of past events, current relationships, and future aspirations.

The transition from cognitive rigidity to suppleness is most evident in the actions taken by veterans post-psychedelic therapy. This adaptability is illuminated through the narratives of those who have steered their lives in new directions—reinvigorating dormant passions, undertaking new educational paths, or embarking on career transitions that once seemed unreachable.

The cognitive flexibility heralded by psychedelic experiences extends into the realms of spirituality and existential understanding. For many veterans, the insights gained are not merely intellectual but deeply spiritual, offering a renewed connection with something greater than themselves. This spiritual awakening often accompanies reevaluating their place in the world, shifting from a sense of alienation to one of interconnection and purpose.

As the psychedelic experience tills the landscape of the mind, a new cognitive ecology emerges—one characterized by resilience, adaptability, and openness. This fertile ground becomes a foundation for lifelong learning and psychological flexibility, allowing veterans to approach life's complexities not as insurmountable obstacles but as opportunities for continued growth and development.

Cognitive flexibility after a psychedelic awakening is akin to discovering a new language with which to engage with the world. It is a language that allows for more nuanced dialogue with one's own experiences and with the experiences of others. For combat veterans, this transformation can be a cornerstone of their healing journey, offering a more malleable and forgiving cognitive framework through which to build a life post-service. The agility gained through this profound cognitive and spiritual expansion paves the way for a future that honors the full spectrum of humanity.

The Altered Landscape of Diagnosis

The encounter with psychedelics ushers combat veterans into an altered landscape, where the rigid labels of clinical diagnoses yield a more fluid and dynamic understanding of their psychological state. This transformative vista offers a fresh perspective on PTSD and moral injury, marking a shift from a purely pathological view to one that is integrative and growth-oriented.

Through the lens of psychedelic insight, PTSD is re-envisioned not solely as a disorder with symptoms to be managed but as a signpost pointing toward a deeper excavation of the self. Veterans report that within the depths of their psychedelic journeys, they encounter a narrative of endurance and wisdom that recasts their traumas as conduits of personal evolution. This perspective seeds a profound sense of purpose. It places their experiences into a context of learning and transcendence beyond traditional views of dysfunction.

Psychedelic experiences often propel veterans beyond the static notion of 'having PTSD' to a more nuanced narrative where trauma becomes a chapter in a larger story of self-discovery. This recontextualization involves remapping traumatic memories and integrating them into a continuous life narrative. Veterans describe a process where fragmented and distressing memories of past events begin to mold together in a way that acknowledges the pain while recognizing the individual's capacity for survival and meaning-making.

The therapeutic work post-psychedelic experience focuses on re-inforcing this cohesive narrative. It encourages veterans to embrace a reconstructed identity that includes their trauma as a pivotal element of their life's journey, not as a defining endpoint. This approach fosters a transformed relationship with their trauma, wherein veterans can view their experiences as integral to their personal growth and self-concept.

In moving from a fractured to an integrated narrative, the veterans' stories of trauma are not erased but are instead imbued with new inter-pretations. By reframing their traumatic experiences within the context of a more significant journey, veterans begin to find a semblance of peace and acceptance. The acknowledgment of trauma as a part of their story allows for a reduction in its power to dominate their sense of self and life narrative.

This section of the book will address these narratives, showcasing how the shift in perception brought about by psychedelic experiences can drastically alter the relationship veterans have with their diagnoses. We will explore how such a profound re-examination of their internal landscape can lead to a holistic healing process that recognizes the multi-faceted nature of trauma and its role in shaping, but not defining, the veteran's identity and place in the world.

Building on the altered perception of diagnosis, the psychedelic journey brings into focus the concept of moral injury—a wound fester-ing not in the flesh but within the soul of a veteran. It's a breach in the very fiber of their moral universe, often sustained when actions taken in the theatre of war clash violently with their fundamental ethical beliefs. This section explores the healing of moral injuries through the prism of psychedelics.

Moral injury, distinct yet entwined with PTSD, requires navigation of the interior landscape where veterans confront actions that once seemed irreconcilable with their values. Psychedelics serve as a compass in this inward expedition, providing directional clarity by dissolving rigid self-judgments and facilitating a reorientation of moral and ethical coordinates. The recalibration often emerges from profound psychedelic insights that underscore the universal connectedness of all beings —an idea resonant with the tenets of Eastern philosophies.

Psychedelics open the gateway to a liminal space where veterans encounter their shadow selves—those parts concealed in the darkness of guilt, shame, and regret. This meeting with the shadow, often illuminated by the light of psychedelic experiences, initiates a dialogue with one's conscience, revealing the full spectrum of one's humanity, which includes fallibility and vulnerability. It is within this honest confrontation that the seeds of forgiveness are sown.

Forgiveness in this context is a radical act of understanding and acceptance, deeply personal yet universally empathetic. The narratives detailed here will include transformative accounts from veterans who, through the psychedelic journey, have been able to extend forgiveness to themselves. They have reframed their perceived moral failings as human reactions under extreme circumstances, shifting their inner narratives from condemnation to compassion.

The cathartic experience of confronting and forgiving one's shadow self is not the culmination of the journey but a passage to ongoing growth. It is reported that many veterans return from the depths of their psychedelic encounters carrying a renewed sense of ethical responsibility and morality. The ramifications of this ethical rebirth are profound, influencing veterans in their daily lives as they make decisions and interact with others through a lens of increased mindfulness and compassion.

Anxiety, Depression, and Substance Use in the Afterglow

In the wake of a psychedelic experience, combat veterans often find themselves in a delicate state of recalibration, navigating the contours of what many describe as the 'afterglow'—a period marked by an acute sensitivity to their internal and external worlds. This phase can bring to the surface emotions and conditions like anxiety and depression, but within this vulnerability often lies a transformative potential. This section will reflect on how, within this afterglow, the shadows of anxiety and depression can be recast through a prism of hope.

Psychedelics have been shown to engender moments of profound clarity and emotional release, offering veterans a vantage point from which despair can be viewed not as an inescapable chasm but as a transient state that has the potential to be traversed with renewed purpose and vitality.

We'll share illustrative narratives that articulate this shift—how an encounter with psychedelics can illuminate the entrenched patterns of thought that often underpin anxiety and depression, providing an impetus for profound changes.

Turning to the relationship with substances, many veterans grappling with addiction find in psychedelics a means to redefine their struggle. Here, the battle is not waged with sheer willpower or stringent self-control, which often spirals into a cycle of guilt and relapse. Instead, it is framed as self-liberation. The narratives will delve into personal accounts where psychedelics have facilitated a profound reconnection with the self, unshackling the chains of substance dependency and laying the foundation for a new relationship with one's own pain and pleasure centers.

This section serves as a pivotal point in the larger narrative, a bridge between the internal reconciliation of moral injury and the complexities of self-forgiveness that follow. We will discuss the influence of psychedelics in altering the course of a veteran's battle with mental health challenges. This chapter will touch upon how this altered state can catalyze long-term change, addressing the underlying causes of anxiety, depression, and substance use disorders.

Integration and the Path Forward

As we transition from the initial afterglow to the long-term journey of integration, the focus shifts to the practical application of the insights gained from psychedelic experiences. Integration is the process of weaving the profound lessons of psychedelics into the fabric of daily life. This task requires patience, persistence, and a nurturing environment.

Self-forgiveness, a crucial aspect of integration, involves acknowledging past actions and their impact without ongoing self-retribution. This path can be complex as it challenges veterans to maintain the delicate balance between accountability and compassion. The integration phase is where the true test of the psychedelic experience lies—the ability to carry forward the sense of interconnectedness, forgiveness, and ethical reawakening into every action and decision.

Integration stands as a beacon for those navigating the profound aftermath of psychedelic-assisted psychotherapy. It's a critical phase where combat veterans stitch together the wisdom gleaned from altered states into the quilt of their everyday lives. Yet, this phase extends beyond mere assimilation of experiences; it demands a rebirth of identity, a reconfiguration of beliefs, and the adoption of a life narrative that embraces growth and understanding.

Self-forgiveness is the first gate veterans must pass on this journey. This is not a mere acknowledgment of the past but an active process of releasing oneself from the shackles of self-condemnation. It requires a profound courage to face oneself, to understand the context of actions, and to acknowledge humanity. This self-forgiveness is not an end but a beginning—a platform from which veterans can launch into deep healing and personal evolution.

This section will explore the multifaceted nature of self-forgiveness, examining how it affects a veteran's life, from self-concept to social relationships. We will present narratives demonstrating how the internal work of self-forgiveness extends outward, influencing relationships with loved ones and re-engagement with the broader community. These stories will reveal the intricate interplay between personal transformation and societal reintegration, illustrating the potential for psychedelics to mend and renew the spirit.

Strategies for successful integration are as varied as the individuals undertaking them. However, common threads of self-reflection, community support, and sustained therapeutic engagement are recurrent themes. We will provide practical guidance on cultivating these strategies, fostering resilience, and continuously applying psychedelic insights. The emphasis here is on establishing consistent practices such as meditation, journaling, and community connection, which ground the veteran's experience and facilitate the translation of psychedelic wisdom into lasting change.

Veterans' narratives will serve as milestones, marking the path of integration as one that can lead away from recurrent anxiety, depression, and substance use. Through the shared wisdom of these stories, we will uncover how mindfulness and interconnectedness can act as shields against the resurgence of mental health challenges.

Moreover, we will discuss the importance of structured integration programs, which provide guidance and support as veterans navigate this terrain. The role of trained facilitators, peer support groups, and ongoing psychotherapy will be highlighted as critical components of a successful integration framework. The goal is to create a structure of support that mirrors the multifaceted nature of the individual's experience.

As we draw the narratives to a close, we will focus on the ultimate horizon for veterans on this journey: cultivating an enduring inner peace and a rejuvenated passion for life. This is the promise of integration post-psychedelic therapy. This promise carries the potential for profound personal and societal transformation.

Weaving Insights into the Fabric of Life

As our narrative traverses the intricate integration process, it becomes clear that professional help is beneficial and essential. This guidance helps veterans integrate psychedelic insights into everyday existence. Psychotherapists versed in the unique dialect of psychedelic experiences can help interpret the language of the mind altered by such profound encounters. This translation is crucial, for it turns esoteric lessons into actionable healing strategies.

Veteran communities, too, play an indelible role in this process. Within these brotherhoods and sisterhoods exists a mirrored understanding, a shared language of service and sacrifice that can deeply empathize with the psychedelic journey's revelations. In these communal spaces, integration is a concept and a lived experience, where growth is nurtured through shared stories, collective wisdom, and an unspoken bond of camaraderie.

To sustain the psychedelic spark—that newfound clarity and enlightenment—veterans must adopt practices that keep the flame alive. Mindfulness and meditation offer solace, acting as daily reminders of the interconnectedness revealed in their journeys. Such practices encourage a continuous presence in the moment, a lesson that psychedelics impart with striking intensity.

However, growth does not stop at self-practice; it thrives on knowledge and understanding. Engaging with educational opportunities allows veterans to deepen their insights and foster a broader application of their experiences. Workshops, seminars, and books on related subjects can reinforce the principles learned during their journeys, embedding them further into the veterans' evolving life philosophy.

Embracing the Journey

The journey does not end upon returning from the psychedelic depths; in truth, it is a perennial passage that each veteran navigates with the wisdom of their experiences as their compass. The path forward is a mixture of individual trials and triumphs. It is also a collective expedition enriched by the communal wisdom of those who walk beside them.

Veterans, armed with the insights of their psychedelic voyages, are tasked with the challenge of continual self-discovery and societal contribution. This journey is neither linear nor predictable, yet it holds the promise of a life reclaimed, a purpose rediscovered, and a peace hard-won.

As we close this chapter, let us reflect not merely on the transformation of the individual but on the potential metamorphosis of society. For each veteran who emerges from the shadow of trauma, bearing the light of understanding contributes to a more compassionate, more insightful world. Thus, the call to embrace this journey becomes a call to action—not just for those who have served but for us all. It is a provocation to witness, to support, and ultimately, to be transformed alongside them. Let us move forward with hope and certainty that from the depths of psychedelic introspection, a stronger, more conscious self can emerge, capable of crafting a life not defined by past wounds but by the wisdom of their scars.

CHAPTER 14

Mending the Family Fabric Post-Psychedelic Experience

Within the family unit, an individual's experiences, emotions, and narratives are intertwined, creating a complex network of relationships. When a veteran returns from the profound depths of a psychedelic experience, they integrate a new strand into this network. This vibrant and potent strand is imbued with revelations and insights that can significantly alter the overall pattern of interactions and connections.

The influence of this new strand extends beyond its path; it affects the direction and the resilience of those around it. For the veteran, the end of the psychedelic journey marks the beginning of a new chapter within the familial context. As they reassume their roles and relationships within the family, the wisdom and transformations they bring forth from their inner explorations begin to filter into the collective consciousness of the family, prompting a shared evolution and deeper understanding.

Emerging from the cocoon of psychedelic exploration, the veteran brings back more than altered perceptions. They carry a renewed sense of self, a psyche touched by the ineffable, and often, a heart cracked open by the sheer intensity of what they've encountered.

This emergence can be disorienting for the veteran and for their loved ones. The family may initially struggle to reconcile the person who left with the one who has returned. The veteran may exhibit new behaviors, display shifts in priorities, or even question long-held beliefs that were once foundational to their character. While potentially unsettling, these changes can also catalyze a more authentic, more profound connection within the family.

As the veteran integrates their psychedelic experience, the family dynamic may undergo a subtle yet profound transformation. Shared values may be re-examined. Communication patterns may shift. There may be an increased capacity for empathy and a heightened sensitivity to each other's emotional states. The family unit may begin to operate less as a hierarchy and more as an ecosystem, with each member responsive to the changes within the others.

This evolution is not without its challenges. The family may have to navigate misunderstandings, renegotiate boundaries, and learn to support the veteran in unfamiliar and necessary ways. It is a journey that requires compassion, a willingness to listen, and a commitment to grow together.

The echoes of the veteran's psychedelic journey can be heard in the most mundane moments—a shared laugh that reaches deeper, a silence that speaks volumes, or a conversation that ventures into previously uncharted emotional territories. These echoes can be healing, as they often carry the seeds of newfound understanding and acceptance.

However, the echoes can also resonate with the pain of old wounds now brought to light, demanding attention and care. The family may be called upon to confront issues that have long been buried to engage more honestly and openly with each other.

As the family adjusts to the veteran's transformed inner landscape, they may find that their views on life, each other, and the veteran are shifting. It is as if the psychedelic experience has acted as a catalyst for the veteran's transformation and for a collective awakening within the family.

This shared journey is not merely about supporting veterans; it is about walking alongside them, recognizing that their healing is intertwined with the healing of the family. It is about finding a new equilibrium where each member can thrive, influenced by the profound experience of one of their own.

In this new dynamic, there is potential for a deeper connection, a more resilient bond, and a greater understanding of the veteran's struggles and triumphs. It is a dynamic that acknowledges the complexity of the human psyche and the power of shared experiences to reshape the individual and the family.

How to Support Your Veteran

In the wake of a veteran's return from the profound journey of psychedelic therapy, the family's abode becomes a sanctuary of transformation—a nurturing ground where patience, understanding, and an open heart are the pillars that uphold the new reality. The veteran, bearing the fruits of his journey's labors, steps back into a world that may now seem as intricate and vast as the one they navigated within.

To welcome them is to embrace a silent metamorphosis that unfolds within the home's walls as much as it does within your loved one's psyche. In this delicate space, a family learns to listen anew, to attune to the subtleties of a reborn psyche. They learn to interpret sighs heavy with meaning and to decipher the stories etched in the furrows of a contemplative brow.

This shared journey is not an isolated path but a collective embrace of the veteran's evolving narrative. Through understanding and empathy, the family becomes a healing container where open communication is encouraged and flourishes. A shared language emerges, one that transcends words and is woven through the fabric of daily life—a look, a touch, a shared moment of silence.

In this nurturing environment, the family unit commits to education, learning together the language of the psyche and the transformative power of psychedelics. Workshops, readings, and discussions illuminate the experiences of the veteran, allowing each member to shoulder part of the transformative weight and, in doing so, lighten the collective load.

Professional guidance remains a beacon, with therapists serving not only the veteran but the whole family. Integration therapy becomes a garden of shared growth, where each root strengthens the collective bond. As active participants, the family finds their roles within the healing process—supporting, understanding, and evolving alongside the veteran.

Yet, in this dance of change, patience is the rhythm that guides the steps of each family member. The metamorphosis does not abide by the tick of a clock but follows a deeper, more organic timing. Celebrating milestones becomes a ritual of recognition for the journey undertaken together.

The family, extending their support, reaches outward to connect with others on similar paths. Support groups and community resources become extensions of the family, offering new perspectives and shared experiences that enrich their understanding.

As the veteran explores newfound interests and passions, the family's support is unwavering. Change is supported and embraced, with an understanding that the veteran's growth mirrors the family's capacity for change. This is a healing not delineated by the stark lines of a manual but painted in the broad strokes of love, empathy, and shared humanity.

Within this dynamic, every support act intertwines with the collective healing process. The home becomes a haven for integration, where each member, connected by bonds stronger for their trials, grows together. The veteran's journey, once solitary, now becomes a shared experience—a melody of resilience, understanding, and profound connection.

Healing Together: The Role of Psychedelics in Family Therapy

In the realm of healing, the advent of psychedelics within family therapy settings heralds a new epoch where the frontiers of collective healing are expanding. As therapists integrate these ancient yet newly rediscovered modalities into treatment, families find unique opportunities to heal together—to bridge gaps that once seemed impossible and to gain an understanding and connection that envelopes each member.

Psychedelics, when introduced into the family therapy process, serve as powerful catalysts for transformation. Under the careful orchestration of trained professionals, these substances can guide the family unit into a liminal space—a communal therapeutic realm where the usual defenses dissolve and the walls that compartmentalize individual pain begin to crumble. In this shared sacred space, the family embarks on a profound journey of collective introspection and healing.

The experience of a shared psychedelic session is far from ordinary. It is an orchestrated communion of souls, guided by the intent to heal, understand, and forge a deeper familial connection. The substances act as keys, unlocking the doors to inner worlds, often revealing unspoken pains, unacknowledged strengths, and buried truths. In this vulnerable state, family members can see and be seen by each other in their full humanity. This process can be both humbling and exalting.

As the family navigates this journey, the therapist's role is akin to that of a cartographer and a guide. They provide the map and the compass—the frameworks of understanding and the techniques to navigate the psychological and emotional terrain that the family will encounter. They ensure the experience remains safe, contained, and aligned with therapeutic goals and objectives.

The potential for breakthroughs during these sessions is significant. Psychedelics have a way of piercing through the layers of persona and ego, allowing individuals to interact with one another at the most fundamental level of being. It is common for members to emerge from the experience with a renewed sense of empathy and an unshakable knowledge of their shared human experience. This can pave the way for forgiveness, the release of long-held resentments, and the rekindling of love and connection that may have dimmed under the weight of individual and collective traumas.

However, the role of psychedelics in family therapy is not solely about the shared experiences within the session itself. The true healing continues by integrating these experiences into the family's daily life. Post-session discussions, guided activities, and continued therapy work to cement the insights and emotional breakthroughs that occurred, ensuring they become a part of the family's new narrative.

This integration process can involve setting new intentions for family interactions, developing new communication patterns, and supporting each other in personal and collective growth. It is in these days, weeks, and months following the psychedelic sessions that the family constructs a new edifice of interaction—one built on the foundations of mutual understanding, shared vulnerability, and a collective commitment to support each other.

In embracing the role of psychedelics within family therapy, we acknowledge the untapped potential of these substances to act as agents of healing for individuals and families. This is a journey back to the essence of connection, where the healing of one is inextricably linked to the healing of the whole and where the family unit can emerge intact but renewed, fortified, and infused with a deeper sense of love and purpose.

Shared Psychedelic Voyage

Within the partnership, especially when one's lead has been shaped by the rigors of military life and combat and the solitude of coping with its aftereffects, the introduction of psychedelics can be akin to a new choreography emerging from the depths of the soul. When both members of a couple partake in the transformative journey of psychedelic exploration, they embark on a shared pilgrimage that has the potential to redefine the contours of their relationship.

This mutual voyage into the psyche can dissolve the veils of isolation that trauma and misunderstanding may have woven between partners.

As each individual confronts and embraces their inner world, they gain insight into their being and an empathetic aperture into their partner's soul. This profound empathy transcends cognitive understanding—it is a felt sense, an emotional resonance that can only emerge from walking a mile in each other's psychic moccasins.

In the aftermath of shared psychedelic sessions, partners often discover a newfound grace in their interaction. Miscommunications that once sparked conflict now become opportunities for deeper understanding. The emotional shorthand that couples develop over time is enriched with new symbols and meanings born from the shared language of their journey.

Integrating these experiences into the fabric of their union is delicate and requires intention. It is a period marked by open communication, mutual support, and the shared responsibility of nurturing the seeds of transformation planted during their psychedelic experiences. The role of a skilled therapist is invaluable here, guiding the couple in translating profound revelations into lasting change within their relationship.

This joint transformation can be particularly beneficial when one partner has been a veteran facing the specters of war. In the shared healing space provided by psychedelics, the couple can address the chasm that such experiences may have created. The veteran is not alone in their healing; their partner, too, becomes an ally in the truest sense, intimately familiar with the landscape of healing and recovery.

However, both individuals must approach this journey with mutual consent and a shared readiness. The decision to embark on such a path should be made with thoughtful consideration and with the guidance of professionals who can ensure the safety and efficacy of the experience.

The shared psychedelic journey has the potential to be a rite of passage, a transformational saga that fortifies the bonds of love and partnership. An incredible potential for growth emerges when two people commit to walking and growing together. This is more than a chapter in their individual stories but a confluence of their narratives, creating a shared epic richer and more profound than the sum of its parts.

This segment of *Warriors of the Mind* highlights the immense potential of shared healing in strengthening the deepest human bonds. It illustrates that within a dedicated partnership, the transformative power of psychedelics can turn personal journeys of adversity and change into a shared experience of deeper love and comprehension.

Guidance for Families

As families navigate the often-unfamiliar waters of psychedelic-assisted psychotherapy with their veteran, comprehensive guidance becomes their compass. This journey, while promising profound transformation, is intricate and multi-layered, and families must be equipped with hope and the wisdom to journey safely and effectively.

The first beacon for families is the acquisition of knowledge. Understanding the psychological terrain of psychedelics means comprehending how these substances can affect the mind, emotions, and spirit. It's about grasping the science behind the therapy and the subjective experiences it can engender. This knowledge serves as a light, illuminating the path ahead and helping families anticipate and understand the changes they may witness in their loved ones.

Families must also be prepared for the potential pitfalls. Just as the psychedelic experience can open doors to healing and insight, it can also unearth deep-seated traumas and provoke challenging emotional responses. Families must cultivate an environment of patience and non-judgment, where the veteran feels safe to explore and express these sometimes difficult revelations. In this, the role of a skilled therapist is invaluable. Such a professional can guide the family in supporting the veteran through challenging moments, offering strategies to maintain balance and perspective.

Furthermore, the therapeutic journey should not be walked in isolation. The cultivation of a robust support network is crucial. This network can include peer support groups, other families who have undertaken a similar journey, and professionals who can offer guidance and reassurance. Families can share their experiences through this community, draw on collective wisdom, and find solace in knowing they are not alone.

The transformative potential of psychedelic-assisted psychotherapy is immense, and families must approach it with both reverence and a proactive stance. They should be encouraged to participate in their therapeutic work, as this can enhance the family's ability to grow and adapt to the changes that the veteran is experiencing. This might include family therapy sessions, where members can learn to communicate more effectively, process shared emotions, and reinforce the family's bonds.

In addition, families should be informed about the integration process—the critical time following the psychedelic sessions when the veteran seeks to incorporate their insights and revelations into everyday life. This period is often where the true healing crystallizes, as the veteran works to align their outer life with their renewed inner landscape. Families play a pivotal role in this process, offering a consistent and loving presence to help ground the veteran's experience.

As their collective journey unfolds, families are encouraged to embrace both the challenges and the gifts that come with psychedelic-assisted psychotherapy. With professional guidance, an understanding heart, and an unwavering commitment to the journey, they can help their veteran incorporate insights from the depths of the psyche into their daily life, fostering healing, growth, and a deeper family connection.

Narrative: A Family's Illustrative Journey

The narrative of the Smith family is suggestive of the transformative power of psychedelic-assisted psychotherapy for the individual and the entire family system. John Smith, the family's cornerstone, returned from his journey within bearing medals of honor from his time in combat but also carrying the gentle embers of hope reignited by his therapeutic experience.

The changes within John were not seismic shifts that rattled the foundations of their home life but rather like the first subtle hints of spring after a long winter. His eyes, which had once held the hard glint of steel, now seemed to reflect the tranquility of a clear blue sky. The timbre of his voice, previously sharpened by commands and the clamor of conflict, now carried the softer notes of a calm and deliberate thoughtfulness.

The dinner table, which had stood as a silent witness to the family's unspoken tensions, transformed into a place of communion and warmth. Here, John unfurled the narrative of his psyche—not as a distant observer recounting facts but as a poet sharing his epic, inviting his family into the landscape of his mind with every word.

His children, who had learned to tread lightly in the presence of his invisible burdens, now stepped closer, drawn by the light of his vulnerability. They began to perceive him not as an enigmatic figure sculpted by the rigors of war but as a father with a canvas of experiences rich in color and depth. They discovered the contours of his humanity, etched with the scars and wisdom his journey had bestowed upon him.

Mary, John's partner in life and the silent bearer of the family's emotional anchor, found herself navigating a new relationship with her husband. The chasm that had stretched between them, filled with the echoes of lost conversations and the chill of intimacy unshared, began to close. They found themselves speaking and truly communicating, embarking on the tender journey of healing the quiet lacerations of years of emotional estrangement.

Like the stories John shared, the Smith family's path was not a straight line from darkness to light. It was a path that zigzagged through understanding and setback, moments of clarity and periods of doubt. But each step forward was a step taken together, a delicate dance of reconnection and rediscovery.

For the Smiths, and indeed for any family grappling with the aftermath of trauma and transformation, the journey is a collage of moments —some fraught with old pain, others alight with new understanding. It's a journey that asks each member to be both a teacher and a student, learning the language of healing and speaking the words of forgiveness.

Ultimately, the Smith family's illustrative journey provokes a question beyond their narrative: What does it mean to be a family in the wake of profound change? Their story suggests that it is not merely about coexisting or surviving but about evolving together—about finding within the depths of shared experience a renewed vision of what it means to love, support, and grow as a collective, forever changed, yet unbreakably united.

CHAPTER 15

The Path Forward After Psychedelic Experiences

Integration Defined

The healing path for a combat veteran is often long and multi-faceted, akin to navigating uncharted territories. Integration serves as the critical juncture where experiences catalyze transformation. This transformative process begins not amidst the psychedelic journey but in the silent interludes that follow. Integrating is weaving profound insights and transcendental revelations from the psychedelic experience into the very fabric of one's being.

For the veteran, integration represents a thoughtful and intentional effort to manifest the wisdom garnered during altered consciousness. It is a purposeful journey from experiencing the extraordinary to living the ordinary in extraordinary ways. Integration is about transforming moments of epiphany into everyday mindfulness and otherworldly visions into visionary ways of engaging with the world.

At its core, integration is about aligning one's values with actions, aligning one's purpose with daily living, and aligning the self that existed before the psychedelic experience with the self that continues to evolve after it. For those who have served in combat, this alignment can often mean reconciling the past with the present, the inner turmoil with new-found peace, and the solitary pain with communal understanding.

This chapter is designed to act as a compass in this terrain, a guiding light to reveal practical pathways and reflective insights. We will explore how integration is beyond just a mental or psychological exercise but a holistic one, engaging mind, body, and spirit in a concerted effort to apply the lessons of psychedelic experiences to one's life.

In the following passages, we will offer practical advice, empirical grounding, and thought-provoking wisdom to assist veterans in this crucial phase of their healing journey. We will discuss the vital role of intentionality in the process, the significance of creating a conducive environment for growth, and the importance of a supportive network that upholds and honors the veteran's transformative experiences.

The subsequent sections will delve into the very heart of this process, providing both the philosophical underpinnings and the hands-on strategies that can help veterans not only to integrate but to thrive in their post-psychedelic life journey.

Strategies for Integration: Creating a quiet or sacred space within the home emerges as an essential sanctuary for reflection and growth in the sacred quest for inner peace and integration. This haven, a physical manifestation of the veteran's need for tranquility and introspection, serves as a personal retreat, where the din of the outside world is hushed, and the soul is given precedence. It can be as simple as a dedicated room corner with comfortable seating, ambient lighting, and perhaps elements of nature, such as plants or a small fountain, to invoke the serene energy of the natural world. Or it might be an area outside, in a garden, or on a porch, where the open sky and earth contribute to a sense of solitude and grounding.

In this space, time slows, breath deepens, and the veteran can engage in the practices that foster continued evolution—be it through meditation, reading, or just being. Here, surrounded by objects that hold personal significance, such as military mementos, family photographs, or tokens from nature, the veteran can create a ritual of reconnection to their inner self, away from the roles and responsibilities that define their daily life. It's a sacred enclave where they can honor their experiences, contemplate their journey, and gently nurture the delicate process of integrating the profound lessons of their psychedelic explorations. This quiet refuge is a physical location and a symbolic gesture of self-care and respect.

As the echoes of the psychedelic journey fade, the process of integration beckons—a time to connect newfound insights with everyday life. This crucial phase begins with structured reflection. Veterans find solace and clarity in the journaling or voice recording ritual, which serves as a vessel to capture the fleeting thoughts, feelings, and revelations that arise post-therapy. This personal chronicle becomes a touchstone for growth, a way to revisit and reinterpret the voyage of the mind with each new reading or listening.

Journaling, a practice as ancient as the written word, serves as a beacon of self-awareness and personal evolution for combat veterans post-psychedelic experience. It's more than a mere diary; it's a ritualistic release, a structured debriefing session after the soul's trudging through the psychedelic landscape. Veterans create a tangible record of their inner transformation by transcribing the often fleeting and elusive visions and emotions onto paper. This log becomes a repository for insights, a way to track progress over time, and a means to decipher the symbolic language of their subconscious.

Regular journaling aids in processing complex feelings and integrating them into a coherent narrative, offering a chance to reflect on personal growth and challenges. Furthermore, this practice can be a therapeutic tool, illuminating patterns of thought and behavior and serving as a silent witness to the veteran's internal battles and victories. Specific prompts such as, "How has my perspective on a particular memory or belief changed since my experience?" or "What insight from my psychedelic journey can I apply to my daily interactions?" can guide veterans in extracting and applying the wisdom gained.

Mindfulness, the art of maintaining a moment-by-moment awareness of our thoughts, feelings, bodily sensations, and surrounding environment, is a cornerstone of integration. Veterans can employ mindfulness to ground themselves in the here and now, often a challenge amid the echoes of past traumas and the uncertainty of civilian life.

Practices can range from formal meditation sessions to mindful eating, walking, or even engaging in conversation with full presence. These exercises train the mind to return to the present, fostering a sense of control and peace. They act as daily touchstones that can help to dissipate the residual fog of war and the intensity of psychedelic experiences. Veterans might start with just a few minutes a day, progressively cultivating a habit that serves as both a shield and compass in their post-service life.

The power of creative expression in the integration process lies in its ability to transmute the ineffable into the tangible. Art becomes a conduit for expression that might otherwise remain locked within. It's a non-verbal language that can express complexities for which words fall short. Engaging in the arts—be it painting, music, sculpture, or writing poetry—can act as a valve, releasing pressure and providing a medium to explore and communicate the psychedelic experience and its aftermath.

These creative pursuits can be particularly valuable for veterans who struggle with traditional communication, providing a solitary and meditative space for self-exploration or a communal one that fosters connection and understanding with others. As veterans pour their internal experiences into their art, they often find that what emerges is a dialogue between their conscious and unconscious minds. This narrative can be shared or held as a private memory to be savored.

There is solace and strength in the company of peers—fellow veterans who share the language of experience. Peer support groups become a collective sanctuary, a place where stories and struggles are shared, understood, and held with respect. This communion is therapeutic, a balm for the soul that affirms one's journey and fosters community and understanding.

The integration path also leads veterans to rediscover their bodies as allies through physical activity. Yoga and tai chi, with their fluid dance between movement and stillness, offer grounding and balance, channeling emotional energy through the discipline of form and the meditation of motion. These practices are exercises and rituals of presence, connecting breath and body moment by moment.

In its boundless wisdom, nature offers a mirror to the tranquility and connectedness once felt in the throes of psychedelic therapy. Time spent under the canopy of trees, beside the rhythm of flowing water, or under the vast expanse of the sky can be both grounding and elevating. The natural world, with its cycles and serenity, reflects the interconnectedness of life, reminding veterans of the harmony they seek to integrate within themselves.

A structured life, punctuated by healthy routines, provides the framework upon which change can be built. Regular sleep, mindful nutrition, and engaging social interactions form a triad of stability, creating the daily backdrop for a life reimagined. Within this structure, veterans find the space to integrate new insights into their waking world, crafting a life that resonates with their transformed inner landscape.

Goal setting transforms the ephemeral into the concrete, translating profound insights into actionable steps. These goals, broken down into achievable milestones, chart a course for positive change.

Educational enrichment complements this personal evolution, as books and resources on psychology, philosophy, and psychedelics offer new lenses through which to view one's experiences. This pursuit of knowledge enriches the mind's soil, fostering a deeper understanding and appreciation of the journey's complexity and transformative power.

For some, spiritual practice intertwines with integration, offering solace and a sense of place within the universe's vastness. Whether through organized religion or personal spirituality, these practices provide a framework that imbues the psychedelic experience with meaning and direction, enriching the veteran's narrative with a transcendent dimension.

Family, too, plays a vital role in this process. Including loved ones in the integration journey fosters mutual understanding and enriches the shared family dynamic. As veterans evolve, so do their relationships, with family members becoming allies and confidants in the quest for understanding and growth.

Professional development might emerge as a newfound calling as veterans seek to align their career paths with their evolving sense of purpose. The insights gained from psychedelic therapy can ignite passions and redirect ambitions, guiding veterans toward vocations that resonate with their transformed sense of identity.

Workshops and retreats offer structured opportunities for deeper exploration, providing veterans with the tools and support to navigate the complex terrain of integration. In these spaces, guided by experienced facilitators, veterans can continue the work of personal development in a community of peers who share the language of transformation.

Throughout this journey, boundaries and self-care remain paramount. Veterans learn that saying no can be as powerful as forging ahead and that self-care sustains the long road of integration. These practices protect and nourish the psyche, ensuring that the veteran can continue to grow from a place of strength and self-compassion.

The process of integration is rich and varied, with each part and process adding to psychedelic insights and experiences. As veterans walk this path, they discover that integration is not a single act but a lifelong journey of becoming an unfolding narrative that honors their service, sacrifice, and continued quest for peace and wholeness.

These strategies are more than mere activities; they are lifelines back to oneself and a place of self-mastery and serenity. They are dynamic practices that can evolve with the veteran, accommodating shifts in healing and new levels of insight. As veterans engage in these practices, they may find that integration is not a static destination but a continuous journey that honors the complexity of their experiences and the depth of their transformation.

Cultivating a Grounded Mindset

The mind's terrain after a psychedelic experience is akin to a landscape after the rain—fresh, renewed, and fertile for new growth. The practices of integration are crucial, but equally important is the soil in which these practices take root—the individual's mindset. A grounded mindset is the bedrock upon which the integration journey is built. It is a mindset that appreciates the gradual unfurling of self-awareness and the incremental nature of personal change. This section will delve into the virtues of patience, self-compassion, and openness to change, which are vital for veterans as they navigate the path of integrating their psychedelic experiences.

Patience is the first cornerstone in cultivating a grounded mindset. Just as one cannot rush to heal a physical wound, we must allow psychological and emotional insights to mature at our own pace. Veterans are encouraged to recognize that integration is not an instant process but a slow and steady journey. The revelations from a psychedelic journey often come in waves, layers that reveal themselves over time, demanding patience to fully understand and assimilate. Patience allows veterans to accept this unfolding without forcing clarity or resolution before its natural time.

Self-compassion is the gentle acknowledgment of one's suffering and the commitment to self-kindness. For many veterans, turning compassion inward can be a challenging shift from the self-discipline and stoicism cultivated in military life. However, in the integration process, self-compassion becomes an act of valor. It is the permission to forgive oneself for past actions and to embrace the present self with all its imperfections. Self-compassion provides a nurturing environment for growth and healing, where setbacks are seen not as failures but as natural elements of the human experience.

Openness to change is the willingness to let go of old narratives and embrace the evolving self. It is an acknowledgment that the mind and spirit, having been touched by the psychedelic experience, are no longer the same. This openness challenges veterans to remain flexible in their self-concept, to question long-held beliefs, and to be willing to re-evaluate their place in the world. It is an invitation to view life as a canvas, ever receptive to new colors and patterns that emerge from the depths of their consciousness.

Cultivating a grounded mindset is to stand firm amid life's flux, to find balance amid change, and to anchor the self in a place of inner strength and calm. It is to view integration as a garden—tending to it requires time, care, and the understanding that not all plants bloom at once. Veterans are encouraged to approach each day with the knowledge that every moment is a step in the process of becoming and that with each step, they grow more into the person they are meant to be. This section implores veterans to honor their journey, nurture their growth with intention, and approach the continuous evolution of the self with courage and grace.

Community and Connection

The transition from combat to civilian life is deeply personal. However, it is a path that need not be trodden in solitude. The community and the bonds of connection provide an essential support system for veterans, especially during the delicate phase of integration post-psychedelic therapy. This network of relationships can become a source of strength, understanding, and validation as the veteran navigates the complex process of integrating psychedelic insights into their daily existence.

In its many forms, the community offers a reflection of the self that can be affirming and transformative. Fellow veterans, sharing the unique language of service and the commonality of their experiences, can offer empathy and camaraderie that transcends words. While each journey is individual, the themes of struggle, growth, and resilience are universal. This shared understanding can significantly lessen the burden of isolation, providing a collective space where healing can be a communal endeavor.

Family members, whose lives are inextricably linked with the veteran, also play a vital role in the integration process. Their support and love can consistently remind the veteran of their worth and potential outside of their military identity. As veterans work to incorporate their psychedelic experiences into their lives, the patience and understanding from family can create a nurturing environment conducive to growth and change. This familial connection, when infused with open communication and a willingness to understand the psychedelic journey, becomes a cornerstone of stability and reassurance for the veteran.

Friends and civilian peers, too, can offer unique perspectives and diverse forms of support. They can provide a sense of normalcy and grounding, offering veterans a view into different ways of life and alternative approaches to common challenges. These relationships can encourage veterans to explore new aspects of their identity, step outside the comfort zones of their previous experiences, and integrate into broader social contexts.

The role of the community in the integration process is multifaceted. It mirrors the veteran's evolving sense of self, reflecting the changes and growth that the individual may not fully recognize. It provides a sounding board for new ideas and a safe space for expressing vulnerabilities. Importantly, community connection also allows veterans to give back and share their insights and support with others, which can reinforce their healing and sense of purpose.

The integration process is an inward journey and an outward engagement with the network of relationships that comprise a veteran's world. This section will explore how veterans can actively cultivate and nurture these connections, finding in them the vital support and recognition needed to foster a true sense of belonging and to fully integrate the profound lessons of their psychedelic experiences into a renewed life in the community.

Psychotherapy's Role

Psychotherapy stands as a beacon for many combat veterans, illuminating the often murky path back to civilian life post-psychedelic therapy. It's a space where the unspoken can find a voice, where the tangled narratives of combat and the vivid tapestries of psychedelic experiences can be unwoven and rewoven into a coherent story. The therapist's office becomes a place of transformation. In this haven, the churning emotions and revelations that emerge from psychedelic therapy can be understood and integrated into the veteran's ongoing narrative.

The role of psychotherapy in the integration process cannot be overstated. Continued engagement with a therapist provides a consistent, supportive framework that veterans can rely on as they process their experiences. This therapeutic alliance allows for a structured exploration of the self. It offers veterans the tools to sift through their memories and insights, make sense of their altered perceptions, and reconcile their past with their present.

A therapist skilled in working with post-psychedelic experiences can guide veterans in contextualizing their journey. They can help identify patterns that may have been revealed during the psychedelic state, assisting in translating profound emotional and spiritual encounters into actionable insights for daily life. This dialogue with a therapist can also provide veterans with a sounding board for their evolving thoughts and feelings, helping validate their experiences and reinforce the positive changes they strive to make.

Moreover, psychotherapy can aid in navigating the emotional turbulence that may follow psychedelic therapy. It is not uncommon for veterans to encounter waves of emotions as they reintegrate into their daily lives, and a therapist can offer strategies for managing these feelings constructively. Whether it's dealing with resurfacing trauma, adjusting to new perspectives on life, or handling the shifts in relationships, the therapeutic relationship provides a compass for steering through these challenges.

The therapeutic environment also offers a space for veterans to practice new skills in a safe setting. Whether developing mindfulness techniques, enhancing communication skills, or exploring new ways of relating to others, the therapist can facilitate growth and learning that supports the veteran's integration journey.

Psychotherapy, in essence, is a partnership—one that honors the veteran's service and experiences while supporting their journey toward healing and wholeness. In this section, we will delve into the myriad ways psychotherapy can serve as an anchor, a guide, and a reflective surface for veterans as they work to integrate the life-altering experiences of psychedelic therapy into a renewed sense of self and a purposeful life path.

As we draw the curtain on Chapter 15, we reflect on the multifaceted journey of integration—a path that requires patience, fortitude, and a commitment to growth. Integration, we've discovered, is not merely a postscript to the psychedelic experience but a continuous, evolving narrative existing throughout every aspect of a veteran's life.

We began by defining the essence of integration, emphasizing its role as the vital bridge between profound psychedelic revelations and the steady rhythm of everyday existence. Within this process, veterans can plant the seeds of insight into the fertile ground of their conscious lives, allowing them to take root and flourish in actions, thoughts, and relationships.

Delving deeper, we outlined strategies that foster this growth: the disciplined reflection of journaling, the anchoring practice of mindfulness, and the liberating act of creative expression. These are not mere tasks but lifelines, each a chapter in the greater novel of the veteran's evolving story.

The necessity of community and connection was highlighted, underscoring that no one is an island, especially not the veteran who seeks to reconcile their internal and external worlds. The support of fellow veterans, the love of family, and the companionship of friends form a network of mirrors and pillars that reflect and uphold the veteran's journey of self-discovery and integration.

Psychotherapy's pivotal role in this process was also illuminated. A structured dialogue with a therapist can serve as a compass through the sometimes-disorienting landscape that follows a psychedelic journey, offering validation, context, and a safe harbor to explore and understand the new contours of the self.

We must remember that integration is an art form, demanding as much from the veteran as any mission once did. It is an act of daily courage to face the ordinary world with a non-ordinary consciousness, to apply the wisdom of profound, sometimes ineffable experiences to the tasks and relationships of daily life. This chapter serves as a guide and an affirmation: the path of integration is walked step by step, with the veteran's inner compass calibrated by the insights gleaned from their psychedelic journey. The road is long, the work demanding, but the rewards are as boundless as the mind and spirit that seek to embark on this transformative path.

CHAPTER 16

Building Resilience & Sustaining Change

Resilience (discussed much in this text) within military life is frequently tied to images of physical endurance and unwavering stoicism. Combat veterans, whose experiences are etched into the very marrow of their beings, often embody this traditional definition of resilience. However, psychedelic-assisted psychotherapy introduces a transformative layer to this concept, reshaping it from a tool of endurance to one of profound evolution.

The therapeutic journey does not simply restore the previous state of being. It catalyzes a renaissance of the psyche. Resilience here is redefined—not as the ability to return to the original form after being bent or compressed but as the capacity to create a new form that incorporates the wisdom gleaned from the depths of one's mind. It is about adopting a more flexible psychological stance that allows veterans to navigate the complexities of civilian life with agility and grace.

As these warriors confront their vulnerabilities through therapy, they harness them as sources of strength. The psychological resilience they build is akin to the physical and strategic resilience cultivated during their military service. It is systematic and deliberate, and a clear-eyed recognition of the self underpins it. The battleground may have shifted from the external to the internal, but the objective remains—to live a life marked by mental clarity and emotional fortitude.

The integration of psychedelic insights facilitates a reorientation of values and priorities. Veterans may explore new career paths that align more closely with their transformed sense of purpose. Others may discover passions and interests previously eclipsed by the demands of service or the shadows of trauma. Relationships, too, may be viewed through a new lens, fostering deeper connections with loved ones and friends. Lifestyle changes become natural extensions of this shift, with veterans gravitating toward activities that nourish both body and soul— through physical fitness, creative expression, or community service.

Moreover, resilience extends beyond individual veterans to encompass their support networks. As they undergo changes in career, lifestyle, and personal interests, their circles of support play a crucial role in sustaining their transformation. These networks—forged in the fires of shared experience—offer resilience, providing a collective strength that reinforces the veteran's journey.

In weaving the threads of resilience through the various aspects of post-military life— psychotherapy, lifestyle, career, and community—a holistic approach to sustaining change emerges. It is a multifaceted resilience that embraces the ability to withstand adversity and to grow from it—to survive and thrive. This is the resilience that psychedelic-assisted psychotherapy aims to instill: a resilience that is dynamic, expansive, and deeply rooted in a renewed sense of self and purpose.

Lifestyle Changes

The path of resilience for veterans is paved with daily practices that extend well beyond the therapy sessions. Lifestyle changes are the bedrock upon which long-term mental health is built, shaped, and solidified. Mindfulness and meditation, once relegated to the peripheries of Western therapeutic practices, now stand at the forefront of psychological resilience strategies, substantiated by a burgeoning body of empirical evidence.

Mindfulness, in its essence, is the practice of being present in the moment without judgment. For the veteran, this practice is a beacon in the often tumultuous transition to civilian life, providing a tool to navigate the ebb and flow of psychological tides. It cultivates a space of awareness, allowing one to observe one's thoughts and feelings with detachment and compassion. This practice is not passive; it actively engages with the inner self, fostering a sense of calm and clarity that can fortify the mind against daily stresses.

Meditation deepens this practice, offering a structured approach to cultivating inner peace. The research is compelling: a consistent meditation routine has been shown to not only reduce the symptoms of anxiety and depression but also to improve attention, concentration, and overall psychological well-being (Jha, Krompinger, & Baime, 2007). For many veterans, meditation becomes a daily touchstone, a ritual that centers and prepares them for the day ahead.

Physical activity complements these mindful practices, serving as a critical component of a resilient lifestyle. The structured discipline of exercise can resonate with the military experience, providing a familiar routine in a new context. The benefits are multifaceted: beyond the well-documented mental health improvements, regular physical activity fosters a sense of accomplishment, reinforces self-efficacy, and can even serve as a social conduit, connecting veterans with peers and communities.

The narrative of Sergeant Johnson is a compelling illustration of these principles in action. Following his journey through therapy, he embraced the discipline of daily runs and the solace of meditation as integral parts of his life. This dual commitment to body and mind provided him with a framework for resilience that was both robust and flexible, capable of adapting to the evolving challenges of post-service life.

The transformative potential of lifestyle changes is not limited to these practices alone. Nutrition, sleep hygiene, and social engagement are critical elements that significantly influence mental health and resilience. A balanced diet can impact mood and energy levels, while adequate sleep is essential for cognitive function and emotional regulation. Social engagement, particularly in meaningful and fulfilling activities, can reinforce a sense of purpose and connection.

By incorporating together mindfulness, meditation, physical activity, nutrition, sleep, and social interaction, veterans can create a comprehensive lifestyle that supports and sustains the profound changes initiated by psychedelic-assisted psychotherapy. It is a holistic approach that acknowledges the intricate interplay between mind, body, and spirit. This synergy can cultivate an enduring resilience capable of weathering life's storms and seizing its joys.

Career Changes

The transformative experiences facilitated by psychedelic-assisted psychotherapy often catalyze a reevaluation of one's career and professional aspirations. This reassessment can be challenging and liberating for veterans, who may have defined themselves mainly through military service. Career changes post-therapy represent a deeper shift toward work congruent with their evolving identity and values.

Many veterans discover their therapeutic journey has profoundly affected their sense of purpose. A career is no longer just a means to an end but a platform for continued growth and self-expression. This could mean transitioning to roles emphasizing service and community leveraging the leadership and teamwork skills learned in the military. For others, it might involve pursuing work that offers peace and fulfillment, such as roles in nature conservation, the arts, or education.

The skills and disciplines acquired in the military are assets in the civilian workforce. Veterans are often adept at leadership, strategy, and operating effectively under pressure—highly valued qualities in many professional settings. Psychedelic therapy can help in reframing these abilities, highlighting how they can be applied in new and diverse fields. By drawing on their unique experiences and perspectives, veterans can carve out niches that capitalize on their strengths and promote personal satisfaction and societal contribution.

Navigating a career change can be daunting. Here, the support systems that veterans have cultivated—peer networks, family, and professional mentors—become invaluable. These networks can offer guidance, opportunities for retraining, and the emotional support necessary during this transition period. Workshops and retreats can provide the tools and confidence to explore new professional avenues.

Despite the growth potential, career transitions can be fraught with barriers, from practical considerations like financial stability to the psychological impact of leaving a familiar role. Acknowledging these challenges while recognizing the opportunities that change brings is essential. Veterans who have undergone psychedelic therapy may find themselves better equipped to handle these barriers, possessing a heightened awareness of their resilience and a clearer vision of their goals.

The benefits of finding the right career path extend beyond the individual. Job satisfaction can improve mental health, work-life balance, and positive social relationships. When veterans embark on careers that resonate with their values and aspirations, the positive effects can ripple, impacting their families, communities, and the broader social fabric.

In constructing the next chapter of their lives, veterans are not just changing jobs but engaging in a profound act of self-realization. Career changes, guided by the deep introspection and personal insights gained from psychedelic therapy, can be a powerful vehicle for continued healing and growth.

Changes in Interest and Passions

The journey through psychedelic-assisted psychotherapy often leads to a renaissance of the self, where old passions may be reignited and new interests discovered. For veterans, this awakening can signal a departure from life once strictly regimented by the demands of military service, guiding them toward pursuits that enrich their spirits and enliven their curiosity.

As the dust settles post-therapy, veterans may find themselves drawn to activities and subjects that they either left behind or never had the opportunity to explore. The deep introspection facilitated by psychedelics can remove mental barriers and inspire a pursuit of passions that align with their transformed sense of identity. Some may turn to creative expressions such as painting, writing, or music, finding solace and joy in the act of creation. Others might be captivated by the natural world, engaging in outdoor activities like hiking, gardening, or conservation work.

Engaging with one's passions has therapeutic benefits, serving as a form of self-care and an extension of the healing process. Activities that foster a state of 'flow'—where individuals become fully immersed and focused on their actions—can lead to increased happiness, reduced stress levels, and a sense of accomplishment. Veterans can harness these activities as hobbies and integral components of a balanced and fulfilling life.

The shift in perspective that comes from psychedelic experiences can renew a sense of wonder about the world. This curiosity can drive veterans toward lifelong learning, whether picking up new skills, returning to school, or simply educating themselves about topics of interest. Pursuing knowledge and skill can provide a sense of progression and fulfillment that supports their overall well-being.

Interests and passions also offer a powerful avenue for social connection and community building. Veterans may find camaraderie and support by joining clubs, groups, or classes related to their interests. Sharing their passions with others helps build new relationships and provides a sense of contribution and belonging.

While new interests can be exciting and invigorating, veterans must balance them with previous commitments and relationships. This balance ensures that pursuing new passions complements rather than conflicts with existing responsibilities and connections. It's about integrating these changes to enhance the veteran's life and relationships.

Ultimately, changes in interests and passions are about allowing oneself to explore and grow. They are about honoring the inner changes that have occurred and allowing those changes to manifest in all areas of life. For veterans, this may mean stepping out of their comfort zones and embracing the unknown enthusiastically and openly.

The evolution of interests and passions, much like the other aspects of change post-psychedelic therapy, is not a linear journey. It is a dynamic process of exploration, learning, and growth. As veterans navigate this journey, they enrich their lives and bring new energies and insights to their interactions with others, contributing to a richer, more diverse community.

Community Support

The power of community in the healing journey of veterans is a force that both anchors and propels. In the aftermath of psychedelic-assisted psychotherapy, when the echoes of transformative experiences still resonate within, the presence of a supportive community becomes crucial. The wisdom of the adage "it takes a village" is never more evident than in the pursuit of sustained therapeutic change.

Support networks for veterans often function as the bridge between the solitary experience of healing and the collective journey of growth. These networks, composed of fellow veterans, family members, and caregivers, provide a space where the language of shared experiences is deeply understood. They serve not only as a sounding board for personal stories but also as a reflective surface where individuals see their experiences in the context of a larger narrative.

The shared struggle and the common bond of service create a foundation upon which veterans can build a renewed sense of self. In these communities, there is no need to translate the language of war, loss, or the struggle for reintegration. Each member is a witness to the other's journey, offering validation and understanding that can only come from having walked a similar path.

Within the supportive framework of these communities, storytelling becomes a powerful tool for healing. The author's retreat experiences, such as with Mission Within, facilitated by the SEAL Future Foundation, are tributes to the profound impact of sharing one's journey. In the sharing, narratives of personal struggle are transformed into stories of collective strength. These accounts, rich with the authenticity of lived experience, serve as beacons of hope and emblems of resilience.

When veterans gather, and narratives unfold, everyone's story becomes part of a greater saga of survival and adaptation. These stories are imbued with the power to comfort, inspire, and forge solidarity bonds. They remind veterans that they are not alone in their journey and that their experiences, while uniquely their own, are part of a shared human experience.

The empathy that flows within these groups is a dynamic and healing force. It creates an environment where vulnerability is not a weakness but a courageous step toward connection and understanding. Empathy fuels the group's resilience, providing a source of strength for members during challenging times. The support network becomes a wellspring of communal fortitude that bolsters the individual's capacity to cope with the ups and downs of post-therapy life.

The impact of community support extends far beyond individual therapy sessions and group meetings. It permeates the day-to-day lives of veterans, offering a constant reminder that they are part of a collective endeavor. The supportive network functions as an extended family that understands the intricacies of the healing process and offers a sustained presence through the various reintegration phases.

Many veterans find that community service is a form of support and healing. By contributing to the welfare of others, they reinforce their sense of purpose and community. These acts of service allow veterans to step into mentorship and leadership roles, supporting others while reinforcing their resilience.

The long-term benefits of community support are profound. As veterans navigate the waters of change, their support networks remain constantly evolving. These connections can last a lifetime, providing an enduring sense of belonging and a persistent reminder of the progress and the journey ahead.

Within the community, each supportive connection is essential. In this supportive structure, veterans find the strength to continue their journey of healing, buoyed by the support of those who understand, care, and stand with them in solidarity.

Veteran Voices

In the chorus of healing, the voices of veterans resonate with a distinct timbre, each a harmonic in the symphony of recovery. These voices, etched with the gravity of experience and the lightness of hope, form the oral history of psychedelic-assisted psychotherapy's impact. They are stories of the resilience of the human spirit.

Lieutenant Miller's story is one of many. It illuminates the path from the depths of PTSD to the peaks of advocacy and support for fellow veterans. His voice joins the chorus of those who have traversed the rugged terrain of the psyche, only to emerge with a message of possibility and renewal. Stories like his create a ripple effect, inspiring other veterans to embark on their journeys toward healing.

Each veteran's story is a unique strand in the broader narrative of change. Some recount a rekindling of family relationships, finding a new capacity for empathy and connection. Others share professional triumphs, discovering careers that resonate with their redefined selves. There are tales of rediscovered hobbies and newfound passions, each birthed from the expansive nature of the therapeutic journey.

The path of healing is seldom linear, and the narratives veterans share often include candid accounts of setbacks. Yet, reframing these moments—not as failures but as integral parts of the journey—underscores the essence of sustained change. Veterans speak of these experiences with a sense of wisdom, recognizing that each obstacle surmounted adds to their reservoir of strength.

At the core of these narratives is a commitment to growth. It is a commitment that endures beyond the therapy sessions, extending into every facet of life. The willingness to grow becomes the North Star guiding principle for veterans as they navigate the complexities of post-therapy existence.

The sharing of these stories is facilitated through various platforms —veterans groups, retreats, public speaking engagements, and publications. Each platform offers a space for veterans to raise their voices, to be heard by a wider audience, and to connect with those who may still be in the throes of their struggles.

The collective narrative that emerges from the amalgamation of individual stories is powerful. It demonstrates the transformative potential of psychedelic-assisted psychotherapy. The collective voice of veterans is a call to action for continued support and research.

In the gathering of voices, the individual and the collective are interdependent. The personal is political, the singular is universal, and the story of one is the story of many. As each veteran speaks their truth, they contribute to a larger dialogue about healing, resilience, and the human capacity for reinvention. These voices collectively tell a story—the ongoing narrative of triumph, challenge, and the unwavering pursuit of growth.

PART V

Family and Friends

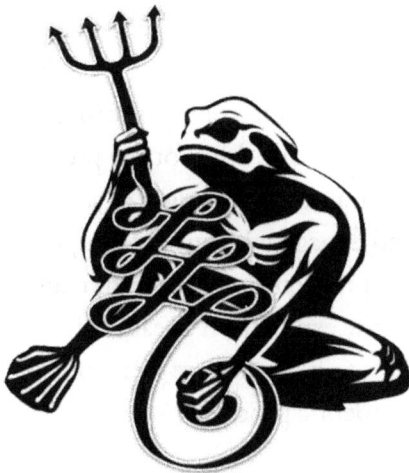

CHAPTER 17

Understanding the Veteran's Journey

When your veteran first enlisted, they stepped into a world that demanded courage, resilience, and a commitment to face the unknown. Now, as they embark on the journey of psychedelic-assisted psychotherapy, these same qualities are called upon once more. However, This time, the battlefield is internal, and the mission is healing and self-discovery. They have transitioned from being a battel-hardened combatant to a warrior of the mind.

Just as enlistment began with a call to serve beyond oneself, engaging in psychedelic therapy signals a call to delve within. The same bravery that propelled them into service is now channeled into confronting inner adversaries and traumas. In both instances, the journey begins with a profound decision to face uncertainty, venture into realms that others may never see, and endure hardships for the promise of a greater good.

Your veteran once trained for the rigor of service, learning to navigate complex terrains and engage with unwavering focus. Psychedelic therapy requires a similar preparation, as veterans ready themselves mentally and emotionally for the exploration ahead. It is a different kind of boot camp, where the skills to be honed are introspection, vulnerability, and openness to the therapeutic process.

Like the comrades-in-arms who stood shoulder to shoulder with them during their service, your role is now a confidant in their psychological exploration and a beacon of guidance. Where once you may have provided support through letters, care packages, or words of encouragement during deployments, now your support is in understanding, patience, and holding space for the shifts that will come.

In the quiet sanctuary of your support, your veteran embarks upon a journey through the turbulent seas of their psyche, a journey as daunting as any faced on the battlefield. Your role in this delicate voyage cannot be overstated, for you must shine a steady light—a beacon of constancy and hope.

Imagine yourself as the lighthouse keeper. You do not wade into the stormy waters to steer the ship; instead, you ensure that your light is visible from afar, a signal that guides the sailor through the night. Your presence, unwavering and reliable, speaks to your commitment. It is felt in the quiet moments, the gentle reassurance of your continued care, and the strength you lend simply by being there.

As the keeper of this light, your guidance is subtle and profound. It is not a hand that reaches out to pull the veteran in one direction or another but a soft glow that illuminates the possibilities in their path. The warm light beckons them toward discovery and understanding, allowing them to chart their course through the healing process.

Safety is a gift you offer—not the safety of never facing the storm, but the promise of a haven once the storm has passed. In your eyes, they must see the reflection of a sanctuary, a place where the tumult of their journey can be laid to rest, where the secrets of their heart can be unveiled without fear. Your solidarity provides a fortress of trust and confidentiality, where their vulnerability is met with unwavering acceptance.

And above all, you are the embodiment of patience. Your steadfast gaze upon the horizon understands that the journey of healing does not heed the ticking of clocks or the turning of calendar pages. It unfolds in its own time, and you stand ready to celebrate each forward step, no matter how small, and to sit in peaceful silence when the soul requires stillness.

Your support is the quiet strength that undergirds the veteran's voyage, the constant light that reminds them that they are not lost at sea even in the darkest night. As they navigate the internal landscapes revealed through psychedelic-assisted psychotherapy, your role is less about the distance covered and more about the promise that every night, there will come a dawn. You will be there to witness it with them.

While embarked upon individually, this journey will touch all who are connected to the veteran. It is a shared voyage in many ways, with your experiences and emotions reflecting the ebb and flow of the veteran's therapeutic process. You will witness the unfolding of a person delving into profound depths to surface treasures of self-discovery and healing—treasures that have the power to enrich life and the lives of all who stand by them.

Veteran will find that the therapy will present in stages, each with its own experiences and challenges. In these stages—each a unique blend of reflection, confrontation, and growth—the veteran will understand the contours of their inner landscape and begin integrating their profound experiences into the fabric of their daily existence. This integration is where the true transformation occurs and where you will play a pivotal role as their confidant and guide.

With this understanding of your role and the courage it takes for your veteran to embark on this voyage, let us now explore the stages of therapy in greater detail, providing you with the insight and empathy necessary to navigate these waters together.

The Stages of Therapy

As discussed thoroughly in this book, psychedelic-assisted therapy is a beacon in the fog for many veterans. As stated, it is not a cure-all but rather a systematic expedition with distinct phases:

Preparation: Before the therapy begins, there is a period of preparation. This is a time for mental and emotional armament as the veteran prepares to delve into the psyche's complex terrain. They are often counseled on what to expect, how to let go of resistance, and the importance of openness to the therapeutic process.

The Psychedelic Experience: Under the guidance of therapists, the veterans enter the core of the therapy. The psychedelic experience can be a labyrinth of the mind, where one confronts the Minotaur of their traumas. In these moments, the veteran might experience a reawakening, an altered state of consciousness that sheds new light on old scars.

Integration: The insights gleaned from the psychedelic experiences are like precious gems retrieved from a deep dive—they must be carefully integrated into the veteran's life. This phase is where the practical magic happens, as veterans apply their newfound perspectives to everyday situations.

The Chrysalis of Transformation

In the heart of the transformation, the cocoon symbolizes metamorphosis for the veteran. It is a sacred space where the constructs of time and identity merge and mingle. Within this chrysalis, the veteran exists in profound liminality, akin to Schrödinger's theoretical cat— simultaneously embodying the past, present, and future. It is a deep paradox where they are both the soldier they once were, the civilian they are now, and the healed individual they are becoming.

Like the enigma of Schrödinger's cat, which is alive and dead until observed, the veteran in the cocoon of transformation is suspended in a state of being that defies simple categorization. They are at once the embodiment of their past experiences and the architect of their future, yet in a state where these timelines converge, neither is fully visible nor defined. It is where past behaviors and identities dissolve, and new possibilities are born, fluid and unfixed.

This stage of transformation is marked by an intense interplay of what was, what is, and what could be. Behaviors and thought patterns that were once automatic may now clash with emerging perspectives, creating a dissonance that the veteran and those surrounding them feel. It's a delicate dance where long-held routines may suddenly seem foreign while new habits are still taking root.

The cocoon is not a void but a vibrant canvas where every hue and stroke of the veteran's life is present. The psychedelics act as a catalyst, not by erasing the past but by infusing it with new meaning. They lay the groundwork for evolution, yet within this chrysalis, the entirety of the veteran's life story—the traumas, the joys, the defeats, and the victories—remains. Every thought pattern and behavior cultivated over a lifetime is present here, swirling in a dynamic interplay of transformation.

It is essential to navigate this stage with mindfulness and grace. For all its growth potential, the cocoon can also be a place of vulnerability. Emerging behaviors and thought patterns may not fit seamlessly with old ones, and this friction can create confusion and uncertainty. As loved ones, it is vital to hold space for this process, recognizing that the chrysalis stage is a natural and necessary precursor to the emergence of a transformed self.

The challenge for the veteran and their loved ones is embracing this transformation's fluid nature. It is to accept that the person within the cocoon is not static but is constantly evolving, shedding old skins, and embracing new forms. It is a time of profound rebirth, where what was once solid and known melts into the potential of what is yet to come.

As we support our veterans through this delicate phase of their journey, we must be prepared for the ebb and flow of transformation. We must be patient as the chrysalis trembles with the stirrings of new life and stand ready to welcome the person who will emerge, knowing they are shaped by every moment they have lived, every battle they have faced, and every dream they dare to chase.

The stones of forgiveness and acceptance often pave the healing road for a veteran. These are not merely destinations but terrains to be traveled, with each step revealing new vistas of the self and the past.

In the depths of psychedelic-assisted psychotherapy, veterans may uncover layers of unresolved pain and guilt that have been forged into the foundation of their being. In this context, forgiveness emerges not as a conscious choice but as a gradual awakening, a dawning understanding that the chains of past grievances—both against others and against themselves—can be released.

This kind of forgiveness is not about forgetting or condoning what has happened. It is, instead, an act of profound liberation. The process of untying the knots of blame and resentment has restricted the heart's natural capacity for compassion. It is a recognition that the burdens of the past need not be the anchors of the future.

As forgiveness paves the way, acceptance follows—a quiet affirmation of the self that has endured the storms of trauma. Acceptance is the acknowledgment of one's imperfections and mistakes, coupled with an embrace of one's humanity. It is the realization that the events and actions of the past are mere parts of the larger story of one's life, each contributing to the person they have become.

Acceptance is not resignation; it is a courageous confrontation with reality. It allows the veteran to stand in the present moment to acknowledge the scars without allowing them to dictate their self-worth. In acceptance, healing finds fertile ground as the veteran learns to regard their past not with eyes of judgment but with a spirit of compassion.

Forgiveness and acceptance create potent alchemy within the veteran's soul. They transform the leaden weights of guilt and sorrow into the gold of wisdom and peace. Through these processes, veterans can reclaim their power over their narratives, re-authoring their stories with a voice that speaks not of victimhood but of survival and resilience.

For loved ones, witnessing this transformation can be both heart-rending and uplifting. It calls for a delicate balance of support and space, allowing the veteran to navigate their path to forgiveness and acceptance while knowing they are not alone.

It is essential to recognize that this journey may not be linear or swift. Forgiveness and acceptance are not always ready to be received; they cannot be forced or hurried. They arrive in their own time, like a sunrise that cannot be rushed but is worth every moment of the night's wait.

As you accompany your veteran on this path, remember that your empathy, patience, and unwavering love are the companions that walk alongside forgiveness and acceptance. Together, they are a strong foundation capable of holding the full spectrum of the veterans' experiences as they step forward into a future unshackled by the past.

The Re-Authoring of Self: Redefining Personal Narratives

For the combat veteran, self-identity is often unknowingly attached to the darkness of trauma. This misattribution can become constant reminder of pain, loss, and struggle. Once etched into the marrow of their being, these narratives have shaped their view of the world and their place within it. Psychedelic-assisted psychotherapy presents an opportunity to reveal the scars of battle and expose the spaces in between—areas of untold strength, resilience, and hope.

The intervention of psychedelics, coupled with the guidance of a skilled therapist, can act as a lens, bringing into focus the overlooked colors and patterns of their personal stories. This lens does not distort or deny the reality of the past. Instead, it magnifies the hidden strengths that have always been present but may have been overshadowed by the narrative of victimhood.

A remarkable transformation occurs as these new aspects of their story come into view. The narrative shifts from a singular focus on suffering to a recognition of survival. Each moment of endurance, each instance where they continued in the face of adversity, is a sign of enduring strength. The narrative of the self as a survivor who has withstood the trials of combat and the conflicts within begins to take precedence.

In reframing their past, veterans can begin to perceive their experiences not as chains that bind them but as challenges they have navigated. This reframing is not an act of erasure. The pain and the past remain, but their meanings are transformed. They become lessons. They become sources of empathy and the foundations upon which new understandings are built.

Through the process of psychedelic-assisted psychotherapy, veterans often come to a place of profound acknowledgment—an acknowledgment of the incredible resilience that has sustained them, of the growth that has occurred through their suffering. They begin to recognize themselves as more than the sum of their traumas. They see the layers of their character forged in adversity but are defined by much more.

With this redefined narrative comes the key to new possibilities. Veterans may discover new identities obscured by the fog of war and the aftermath of service. They begin to engage with the world not as the person they once believed they were, destined to a life constrained by their experiences, but as individuals capable of change, growth, and renewal.

These shifts in self-perception naturally extend to their relationships with others. As their internal narrative changes, so does their interaction with the world. They may approach relationships with greater openness and vulnerability, willing to share their stories not as tales of sorrow but as epics of survival.

The transformation can be awe-inspiring for those who stand by them—family, friends, loved ones. It requires a willingness to let go of the veteran as you knew them, to embrace the unfolding story, and to support them in the continuous process of becoming. In sharing this new narrative, connections are deepened, understanding is fostered, and healing is shared.

As the veteran re-authors their narrative, they reclaim the pen that writes their future, guided by a hand that is theirs and supported by those who walk the path with them. This re-authoring is a journey that honors the past, cherishes the present, and looks to the future with eyes wide open to the potential within.

Navigating the Shifting Sands of Relationships

In the wake of psychedelic-assisted psychotherapy, the veteran finds themselves on a cusp of transformation, and this personal evolution casts a new light on their relationships, moving from discord to understanding and empathy. Yet, as the hues of their connections change, both veterans and their loved ones must navigate the nuanced terrain that lies ahead.

As the veteran's internal landscape undergoes its metamorphosis, the very essence of their relationships follows suit. It is a delicate dance where steps of progress are interlaced with the potential for missteps. The newfound harmony that begins to resonate within once-strained bonds carries with it the echo of past discord, reminding all involved of the journey that has led them here.

The veteran and their loved ones learn to adjust to each other's rhythms. Once laden with the armor of guardedness, conversations slowly shed their protective layers, revealing the vulnerability of authentic dialogue. This newfound openness is a double-edged sword; it carries the power to heal but also exposes old wounds to the sting of fresh air.

The path of communication becomes a winding road. There are moments when the veteran may retreat into silence, a necessary respite as they sift through the shifting sands of their psyche. In these moments, loved ones learn the value of presence without the insistence of speech, offering a silent solidarity that speaks volumes.

Expectations, those silent overseers of relational dynamics, may also require recalibration. Where loved ones once envisioned a linear progression toward healing, they now understand the journey to be more akin to the ebb and flow of the tides—constant yet unpredictable. They celebrate the small victories, recognizing the planted seeds of more significant triumphs.

As the veteran grapples with the fluidity of their changing self, so must those around them. It is not merely the veteran who must relearn how to navigate the world but also their family and friends. Together, they redraw the boundaries of their interactions, crafting a new map that respects the need for independence and the comfort of intimacy.

Backslides into old patterns are not failures but part of the intricate change process. These are the times when the bonds of relationship are tested and, if met with patience and understanding, can be strengthened. It is a shared journey where the veteran and their loved ones must occasionally falter to find their footing in the new landscape of their connection.

Throughout this transformative process, unwavering, unconditional love holds it all together. This love becomes the constant star of change in the night sky, a fixed point of light that guides the veteran and their loved ones through the darkest hours.

In embracing the veteran's unfolding narrative, their loved ones witness the individual's rebirth and participate in a mutual renaissance of their shared history. They learn that transformation is not a destination to be reached but a path to be walked together, step by step, with courage, grace, and confidence from knowing that no matter how the sands may shift beneath them, they will not walk alone.

Journeying Through the Landscape of Change

For those who stand alongside the veteran, the transformation induced by psychedelic-assisted psychotherapy is akin to watching the dawn break over a once-familiar landscape, now redefined by the light of a new day. Though laden with hope, the changes bring with them a terrain that is uncharted and unpredictable. It is a path that demands from family and friends a resilience parallel to that of the veteran—a willingness to adapt, to be patient, and to maintain an ever-open dialogue.

As loved ones, you find yourselves as companions in a journey that is not your own yet intimately affecting you. It's a shared space where the joy of witnessing the veteran find new horizons of self-understanding is interspersed with the challenges of adjusting to the shifts in their being. The road may be strewn with setbacks—moments where old patterns resurface, progress seems to falter, and the mists of uncertainty obscure the way forward.

Yet, it is in navigating these very challenges that the potential for deepened connections emerges. Every conversation, shared silence, and tentative step into the newfound emotional landscape becomes an opportunity to fortify your bonds. Through these interactions, you may also find your perspectives broadening, your understanding deepening, and your capacity for empathy expanding.

Embracing this journey requires an acknowledgment that transformation is a perpetual process. It is not a single point on the horizon but a series of continuous steps, each carrying the veteran— and you—forward. As the veteran venture through their inner topography, reshaped by their therapeutic experiences, they find solace in knowing they do not travel alone.

Your role as family and friends is not to chart the course but to walk it alongside them. You are not the guides with the map but the fellow travelers willing to face the unknown together. It is a delicate balance of giving support and allowing space, offering insights while respecting the veteran's wisdom, and sharing the journey without leading it.

In this shared voyage of rediscovery and renewal, remember that every step taken together is a step toward a shared future, where the veteran's healing is interwoven with the collective growth of all who accompany them. You are the witnesses to their transformation, and in turn, you are transformed, each of you contributing to a mutual narrative of resilience and hope.

As the landscape unfolds, with its new contours and vistas, you learn the art of walking in step with change. With each day, with each challenge faced and joy embraced, you are reminded that the journey of transformation—like the bond that ties you to the veteran—is a living, breathing entity, always moving, constantly evolving, always inviting you to discover the beauty in the process of becoming.

Embracing the Language of Transformation

In the aftermath of psychedelic-assisted therapy, veterans often find themselves traversing a new emotional terrain where the familiar signposts of verbal communication may no longer suffice. For the families and friends accompanying them, understanding these changes requires a shift from a problem-solving mindset to one of empathetic companionship. It's a journey of compassionate curiosity, not to unravel a mystery but to be steadfast alongside the veteran's path of self-discovery.

As veterans explore this new landscape, they may discover unique modes of expression that capture the intricacies of their internal experiences more richly than words. Some may turn to the arts, where a paintbrush or a musical note can articulate volumes of emotional depth. Others might find solace in writing, where the cadence of their words, the metaphor in their poetry, or the rhythm in their stories echoes the profound shifts within their psyche.

In these instances, the role of loved ones is to become fluent in these non-verbal languages. To see the silent communication in a veteran's painting as a rich narrative painted in the colors of their soul. To hear the unspoken words in the melody they play or the lyrics they pen—each a pulse of the heart made audible. It's about creating a space where these expressions are welcomed with an open heart and a receptive spirit.

The challenge for those close to the veteran is to resist the urge to impose the familiar structure of verbal dialogue. Instead, it's about learning to understand and appreciate the new forms of connection that emerge. It's about recognizing that sometimes, sitting together in shared silence can be as communicative as a conversation, and standing side by side in front of a canvas can be as connecting as a shared meal.

Navigating post-therapy changes is thus a collective venture. It's about accompanying the veteran on their journey without the expectation of traditional communication. It offers a non-judgmental space where the veteran can explore and express their shifting inner world in whatever form it takes. Loved ones provide a sanctuary of understanding.

In this shared space, the transformation is always an individual endeavor but also a relational one. The veteran's exploration of new forms of expression invites those around them to participate in a deepened communication that goes beyond words. Together, they craft a unique dialect of mutual understanding that honors the veteran's experience and fosters a deeper bond of connection.

This new language of transformation becomes a bridge between worlds, allowing for a profound communion that supports the veteran's healing journey. It underscores the significance of being truly present, the resilience of an open mind, and the unlimited possibilities for connection when we fully engage with every aspect of human emotion.

Illuminating the Path Home

As we draw the curtains on this chapter, we recognize that the journey you are undertaking with your veteran is one of profound significance. It is a commitment that goes beyond mere observation to active participation in the ever-evolving narrative of their life. This journey demands patience, a deep reservoir of empathy, and an enduring belief in their ability to heal and transform.

Understanding your veteran's experience through psychedelic-assisted psychotherapy is akin to learning a new language—one that communicates through the subtle interplay of emotion and insight, often without words. It is a language that speaks of the courage to face the depths of one's psyche and the strength to integrate those revelations into one's life. As loved ones, you become the compassionate listeners, the interpreters of this silent dialogue, and the witnesses to the unfolding miracle of personal renaissance.

Your empathy is the beacon that helps you navigate this journey. With each step and expression of the internal tumult and triumph, your presence offers a consistent source of light and warmth. In this shared space, your veteran is not alone. They are accompanied by your unwavering belief in their potential for renewal—a belief that acts as a powerful catalyst for healing.

As we transition from this foundation of understanding to the actionable terrain of support, remember that your role is invaluable. The subsequent chapters will provide strategies to cultivate an environment where healing, understanding, and mutual growth can flourish. You are not just passive observers but active participants in creating a sanctuary where the veteran can continue to heal.

Your support is a compass guiding your veteran through the occasionally stormy seas of post-therapy adjustment back to the shore of shared experience and connection. It is a support that does not waver with the winds of change but stands firm in commitment and love.

With this understanding, we will explore the practical measures you can take to reinforce this supportive framework. Together, we will discover how to create a space that welcomes the veteran back from their profound inner journey and celebrates and nurtures the growth they bring with them. Your support helps guide your veteran home.

CHAPTER 18

How You Can Help: Support and Communication

To expand on the themes of communication and relational dynamics within the context of providing support to veterans undergoing psychedelic-assisted psychotherapy, we let's delve deeper into the realms of psychological theory, attachment styles, communication models, and evidence-based practices that enhance bonding and practical support. This comprehensive approach will provide a robust framework to understand and improve their supportive roles.

Within the transformative journey of psychedelic-assisted psychotherapy, the nuances of support that friends and family provide are crucial. This chapter delves into the psychological theories and research that underpin effective communication and relational dynamics, aiming to give supporters a comprehensive understanding of how to be there for their veterans in the most impactful ways.

Emotional Intelligence

Emotional intelligence is the research interest of psychologists John D. Mayer and Peter Salovey, later popularized by author Daniel

Goleman. It refers to the capacity to acknowledge, grasp, and manage our emotions and those of others. This nuanced understanding of emotions is particularly crucial when offering support to combat veterans, whose emotional landscapes have been intricately shaped by their unique experiences.

In the context of supporting a combat veteran, especially one who may be processing the aftermath of psychedelic-assisted psychotherapy, emotional intelligence acts as a compass that guides the supporter through the complex terrain of the veteran's feelings and emotional responses. This journey requires a sensitive and informed approach, attuned to the subtleties of the veteran's internal world.

The first step in applying emotional intelligence is recognizing and accurately interpreting both the veteran's and one's emotional states. This recognition goes beyond the superficial labels of "happy" or "sad" to a more sophisticated understanding of the nuances in between. For a veteran, emotions may not always be expressed overtly; they may manifest through a change in posture, a particular look in the eyes, or a shift in tone of voice. The supporter must be vigilant, like a watchful guardian, able to perceive these subtle signs and acknowledge them without rushing to interpretation.

To support a veteran effectively, one must recognize emotions and strive to understand their origins and implications. Combat veterans may experience a complex spectrum of emotions stemming from their service, including pride, grief, guilt, or confusion. Post-therapy emotions can be even more layered as veterans grapple with newfound insights into their psyche. A supporter with high emotional intelligence will seek to comprehend these emotions within the context of the veteran's narrative, recognizing the interconnectedness of past experiences, present struggles, and future anxieties.

Armed with recognition and understanding, the supporter must manage emotions with finesse. This management is not about controlling or stifling emotions but rather about facilitating a space where emotions can be expressed healthily and constructively. For a veteran, articulating complex emotions can be a formidable challenge. Here, the supporter's role is akin to a skilled conductor, gently guiding the veteran toward an emotional expression that fosters healing and growth while ensuring that their emotional responses are supportive and not overwhelming.

Lastly, emotional intelligence involves the ability to use awareness of emotions to inform and guide behavior. Through their understanding, a supporter can help the veteran channel their feelings into positive action or reflection. This might mean encouraging the veteran to engage in activities that provide solace or invigorate them, or it could involve facilitating conversations that allow the veteran to explore the depths of their emotions in a safe and nurturing environment.

In the dance of support and care, emotional intelligence is the music that allows for a fluid and graceful movement between supporter and veteran. It is the language through which unspoken feelings find voice and through which the intricate stories of the heart are told and understood. A supporter's emotional intelligence can shine as a beacon of hope and understanding for the combat veteran, illuminating healing and wholeness.

Psychological Theory and Attachment

Attachment theory emerges as a profound map of our earliest relational blueprints. John Bowlby, the pioneer of this theory, alongside Mary Ainsworth, who furthered his work with her meticulous research, invites us to consider the profound impact of our first bonds—the ones formed in the cradle of childhood—which continue to echo into the corridors of our adult relationships.

These early attachments, characterized by warmth and closeness with our caregivers, are not merely sentimental memories but the silent architects of our relational worlds. They mold our expectations, shape our needs for closeness or space, and color how we reach out or retreat in relationships throughout our lives.

The nuanced understanding of attachment styles—be it the security found in the steady presence of a responsive caregiver, the anxiety of inconsistent nurturing, the avoidance born of emotional unavailability, or the disorganization that follows in the wake of chaos—illuminates the patterns of how we support and seek support. It's as if each style speaks a different dialect of care, expressing and interpreting signals of support in a deeply ingrained manner.

For those who stand beside veterans as they journey through the healing process of psychedelic-assisted psychotherapy, a grasp of these attachment dialects can be transformative. It enables supporters to tune in to the veteran's unique frequency of need and response, understand when to draw close, give space, offer words, and when presence alone suffices.

This empathetic attunement, informed by the knowledge of attachment theory, allows for support that resonates with the veteran's innermost needs.

Communication

For those standing alongside veterans, an awareness of their attachment style and that of the veteran can be enlightening. It can guide the supporter to tailor their approach, particularly as the veteran confronts the vulnerabilities that arise during and after psychedelic therapy.

Recognizing and adapting to these styles can lead to a more nuanced and compelling support that resonates with the veteran's personal experiences and needs.

Within the context of psychedelic-assisted psychotherapy for veterans, support is an art that rests on four foundational pillars drawn from the wisdom of attachment theory. These pillars are not mere concepts but living practices that, when embraced, create a sanctuary for the veteran's unfolding journey of self-discovery and recovery.

The first pillar is security and trust. It is the consistent and reliable presence that a supporter offers, reminiscent of the steadfastness found in a secure childhood attachment. This sense of safety is the soil where veterans can plant their experiences, no matter how tumultuous, and trust that the winds of judgment or misunderstanding will not uproot them. In this secure space, veterans can dare to explore the deepest recesses of their inner world, knowing they are not alone and that there is someone firmly in their corner, unwavering and resolute.

Autonomy is the second pillar, rising like a beacon of respect for the veteran's capacity to navigate their healing journey. It is the gentle encouragement given to veterans to make choices about their path of recovery, to take the helm and steer through their waters. By honoring the veteran's need for self-determination, supporters acknowledge the inherent strength and wisdom residing within everyone. This empowerment is a quiet nod to the veteran's ability to reclaim control over their life narrative, an essential step toward self-efficacy and empowerment.

Then there is empathy, the third pillar, perhaps the most tender. Empathy asks supporters to step out of their shoes and into the veterans, see the world through their eyes, and feel the pulse of their emotions without the slightest hint of judgment. This pillar is not about mere understanding; it's about connection. When a veteran shares their innermost feelings and experiences, particularly those that emerge from the depths touched by psychedelic therapy, they are met with a heart that listens and hands that hold their truths gently. This empathetic embrace is validation in its most profound form, recognizing the veteran's humanity and the authenticity of their experiences.

The fourth and final pillar is validation, the cornerstone of the structure. To validate a veteran's experiences and emotions is to affirm their very existence, to acknowledge the weight of their journey, and to offer a reflection that says, "You are seen, you are heard, you are real." This acknowledgment is not passive; it is an active engagement that can light the flame of healing and growth, illuminating the path forward.

These four pillars—security, autonomy, empathy, and validation—are the guardians of the veteran's healing process. They create a space that is both a fortress against the storms of isolation and a garden where new beginnings can take root. For supporters, these pillars are a call to action, a guide for how to be present in the most meaningful of ways, offering support that is as unwavering as it is compassionate. In embracing these four pillars, the healing journey for veterans becomes a shared pilgrimage. A path walked with those committed to holding the light of understanding and the warmth of connection.

Communication Models in Depth

Effective communication is the cornerstone of providing support to veterans undergoing transformative experiences like psychedelic-assisted psychotherapy. It is a multifaceted endeavor encompassing verbal exchanges, non-verbal cues, emotional intelligence, and contextual awareness. We turn to established models that offer a roadmap for navigating this complex landscape to understand and enhance this communication.

The Transactional Model of Communication plays a melody that resonates deeply with the experience of those offering support to veterans in the aftermath of psychedelic-assisted psychotherapy. Crafted by the insightful minds of Harold H. and Ruth C. Hartley, this model paints a picture of communication not as a simple exchange but as a dynamic, living process where each person is both the artist and the canvas, simultaneously imparting and receiving messages.

As supporters engage with veterans, they step into a dance of dialogue where every gesture, word, and silence is part of a complex choreography. This model does not confine communication to a rigid pathway from one person to another; instead, it acknowledges the fluidity where roles as senders and receivers blur and merge. In this dance, supporters are fully present, giving and taking, in a rhythm that honors the veteran's voice as much as their own.

The dance floor is vast, and the music is nuanced. Feedback is not constrained to the verbal; it flows through the air in the form of a furrowed brow, a gentle nod, or a subtle shift in posture.

These silent notes are as potent as any spoken word, and the supporter who understands this can listen with their eyes and ears, attuning to the unspoken symphony of the veteran's heart.

Within this intricate waltz, the supporter's emotional presence is paramount. To truly hear is to listen deeply to the words and understand the stories they carry, the emotions they're laden with. Active listening becomes a sacred act, a pledge to hold the veteran's words with care and respond not with haste but with thoughtful consideration. It is in this sacred space that messages are felt and understood.

As the melody of communication unfolds, the feedback loop becomes a spiral of growth. Every nod, every shared silence, every empathic response is a step that spirals upward, elevating the quality of interaction. In this space, misunderstandings are gently unraveled, and trust slowly emerges within the conversation.

The setting in which this dance occurs is as varied as the landscapes of the mind. Emotional, social, or environmental context sets the stage for communication pirouettes. The supporter, attuned to the veteran's internal and external world, becomes a skilled choreographer, selecting moments and methods that resonate with the veteran's emotional state and the unique contours of their journey.

In the tender aftermath of therapy, when the veteran's words may fail to capture the depths of their transformation, the non-verbal cues carry the weight of cathedrals. A hand's clasp, the patience in a companion's eyes, the shared breath of quiet companionship—these are the silent languages that speak volumes, the tender gestures that say, "I am here with you," more eloquently than any poetry could aspire to.

Thus, through the lens of the Transactional Model, communication is reimagined as an exquisite tapestry woven from threads of presence, empathy, and understanding, creating a fabric strong enough to hold the complexities of the veteran's experiences and soft enough to comfort their soul. The supporter, embracing the full spectrum of this model, becomes a beacon of connection, guiding the veteran with a light that shines forth from the heart of shared humanity.

As we delve into the area of communication models, it becomes evident how these frameworks can be artfully woven into the supportive care provided to veterans undergoing psychedelic-assisted psychotherapy. Though distinct in their approaches, the Interactive and Constructivist models offer a depth of understanding that can enhance how supporters connect and communicate with veterans on their journey toward healing.

The Interactive Model, emphasizing feedback, transforms conversations into a dance of reciprocity. It's a dynamic interplay where each participant, the supporter, and the veteran take turns leading and following. This model breathes life into dialogues, allowing them to evolve from mere exchanges of words to resonant encounters that can touch the heart and soul. When supporters embody this model, they become mirrors reflecting the words, emotions, and intentions behind them. They offer feedback that is not merely a response but a reflection that helps the veteran see their progress and challenges more clearly.

On the other hand, the Constructivist Model invites us to recognize that we construct our reality based on personal experiences and beliefs. When this understanding is brought into conversations with veterans, supporters become architects of a shared reality. They listen with an awareness that the veteran's perceptions are painted with the unique hues of their experiences, especially following the profound introspection that psychedelic therapy can provoke. Supporters using this model do not impose their reality but seek to understand and respect the veteran's reconstructed world, facilitating a connection deeply rooted in empathy and acceptance.

Through these models, communication transcends its primary function, becoming a therapeutic tool. Supporters learn to create a space where veterans feel seen and heard, a space that acknowledges their reality, however altered it may be by the therapy. It's a space where silence can be as eloquent as words, where a nod or a pause can speak volumes, and where the simple act of being present communicates a commitment to the veteran's journey.

This narrative of support is about conveying messages and building a bridge of understanding that can bear the weight of a veteran's hopes and struggles. It's about constructing a dialogue that is both a shelter and a pathway: a refuge from the storms of confusion and isolation and a path toward shared understanding and deeper connection.

Thus, communication becomes an art form—a medium through which supporters and veterans create a masterpiece of connection, sustaining the veteran's healing process. The supporter, equipped with the insights from these communication models, becomes an artist capable of painting strokes of comfort, solidarity, and understanding on the canvas of the veteran's psyche, guiding them gently toward a horizon of recovery and beyond.

Facilitating Deep Relational Dynamics

In the intricate journey of healing, especially for combat veterans who have bravely navigated the often turbulent waters of psychedelic-assisted psychotherapy, the creation of a robust and nurturing bond with their supporters is not merely beneficial but essential. The foundation of this bond is formed from the mortar of research and evidence-based practices that highlight the critical role of the therapeutic alliance —the relational bridge built on trust, mutual understanding, and the shared commitment to the veteran's well-being.

The alliance, akin to the sacred pact between therapist and client, holds just as much potency when it is between the veteran and their loved ones. It is a pact that is fortified by the very acts of support that loved ones provide: the active listening that tunes in to the veteran's voice with a reverence that elevates their words, the empathetic engagement that recognizes and resonates with the veteran's emotional truths; and the shared understanding that fosters a collaborative spirit in navigating the path to healing.

Within this alliance, reflective listening is the melody that harmonizes the veteran's narrative with the supporter's attentive presence. It is a practice of echoing the words and the essence of what the veteran communicates within the dichotomous, complex spectrums of hope and despair. This reflective process is a silent nod that conveys a deep respect for the veteran's perspective—a validation that can be felt in the soul.

The harmony of this melody is the supporters' emotional intelligence in relational dynamics. It is the attunement to the ebb and flow of the veteran's emotional world, the subtle dance of understanding that moves to the rhythm of shared feelings. When supporters navigate this landscape with an awareness of both their own emotions and those of the veteran, they create a sanctuary where the veteran can find solace and recognition. In this shared emotional space, the veteran is not alone; they are accompanied by a compassionate witness to their innermost experiences.

Adding rhythm to this profound dance of connection are Non-Violent Communication (NVC) principles. This philosophy of interaction infuses compassion into the very heart of dialogue. When supporters adopt NVC, they speak a language that transcends blame and criticism, opting instead for expressions rich with empathy and devoid of judgment. This compassionate discourse opens the gates to vulnerability, allowing the veteran to express needs and emotions in a space that is not only safe but nurturing.

Together, these practices—the deep listening that hears beyond words, the emotional intelligence that feels beyond expressions, and the compassionate communication that speaks beyond the ordinary—create a relational dynamic that is both a shelter in the storm and a garden where growth is cultivated. This dynamic does not just support the veteran; it transforms the nature of support into an art form, where every gesture, every word, and every silence is an act of profound respect and connection.

Through these evidence-based practices, the bond between supporters and veterans becomes a living entity comprised of the healing power of empathy, understanding, and the shared human journey. In this bond, the true essence of support is found—a connection that holds the potential to heal the wounds of combat and celebrate the strength and resilience of the human spirit.

Applying Closeness Research

The quest to cultivate closeness with a combat veteran, especially one on the path of healing from the invisible scars of war, is akin to tending a garden that has seen both neglect and storm. The research on closeness in relationships, particularly the pioneering work of Arthur Aron and his colleagues, sheds light on the delicate art of nurturing this garden, encouraging the growth of intimacy through shared experiences, vulnerability, and mutual discovery.

Aron's research illuminates the path to closeness through activities designed to peel back the layers of superficiality that often cloak our daily interactions. Sharing personal stories is one such activity; it is a way to gently unearth the narratives that have shaped the veteran's life. When shared in a space of mutual respect and attention, these stories can act as a bridge connecting the inner world of the veteran with that of the supporter. Each story reveals a landscape of hopes, dreams, fears, and triumphs, inviting the supporter to enter the veteran's world with a deeper empathy and understanding.

Asking deep, probing questions is the water that nourishes this burgeoning closeness. When asked with genuine curiosity and without judgment, these questions encourage the veteran to delve into their psyche to reflect on their experiences and the meanings they derive from them. This process of inquiry and reflection can catalyze moments of profound insight, not only for the veteran but also for the supporter, as they come to understand the complexities of the veteran's journey on a much deeper level.

Participating in shared challenges is yet another way to foster a sense of unity and intimacy. These challenges can be physical, intellectual, or emotional endeavors that the veteran and supporter undertake together. As they face and navigate these challenges, they build a shared narrative of overcoming and resilience, a narrative that becomes a shared thread in the fabric of their relationship. Striving toward a common goal or overcoming a shared obstacle can forge bonds of closeness that are difficult to replicate in ordinary circumstances.

By weaving together personal storytelling, thoughtful questioning, and joint ventures, closeness becomes an abstract concept and a lived reality. It transforms the relationship into a dynamic space where both the veteran and the supporter can explore the dimensions of their connection, discovering new strengths and facets of each other in the process. This closeness, cultivated with intention and nurtured through shared experiences, becomes a powerful agent of healing, offering the veteran the warmth of companionship and the strength of a bond that transcends the ordinary, providing solace and support on the road to recovery.

Supporting Family Bonds and Bonding

Within familial relationships, where each member's step affects the rhythm of the whole, family systems theory offers profound insights. This theory, which views the family as an interconnected organism rather than a collection of individuals, provides a lens through which we can understand the delicate balance that sustains a family's well-being. For families of combat veterans, this perspective is especially poignant, as the ripples from one member's healing journey can become waves that either unsettle or restore the family dynamic.

When a veteran embarks on the path of recovery, particularly through the intense and introspective experiences of psychedelic-assisted psychotherapy, their transformation does not occur in isolation. Each family member is part of this transformative process, influenced by and contributing to the veteran's healing. Recognizing this interdependence is the first step toward fostering a supportive family environment.

To support this balance, families can engage in practices reinforcing their unity and collective resilience. Open and honest communication becomes the cornerstone, allowing each member to voice their experiences, concerns, and hopes. In this shared communicative space, the family can address the changes they are witnessing within their loved one and the family structure.

Adaptation is also key in supporting family bonds. As the veteran heals and evolves, so too must the family system. This may involve redefining roles, renegotiating boundaries, and finding new ways to connect and support one another. Like a tree, the family must be flexible enough to bend with the winds of change without breaking, finding new strength in their altered form.

Collaborative growth further solidifies these bonds. When families face challenges, they can come together to find solutions that consider the well-being of each member. This could involve family therapy, shared activities, or regular gatherings where everyone can check in and be heard. By growing together, families support the veteran's healing journey and fortify their collective capacity to navigate future challenges.

In the heart of this support system lies empathy. The ability to empathize with the veteran's experiences while extending that understanding to each family member's journey creates a strong and soft support fabric. It is in the moments when empathy is most needed— when a family member feels overwhelmed, when the veteran struggles to articulate their inner transformation, or when the family dynamic shifts —that the true strength of the family bond is tested and solidified.

By integrating the principles of family systems theory into the family's daily life, support for a combat veteran becomes a shared mission. A mission that holds at its core the values of interdependence, communication, adaptability, collaborative growth, and deep empathy. In this mission, the family stands not as a group of individuals but as a unified entity, ready to support one of their own through the trials of healing and into the triumphs of renewed connection and understanding.

Final Thoughts

Let's step back and survey the landscape we've traversed. We've navigated through the dense forests of psychological theories and emerged into the clearing of understanding surrounding the emotional battleground veterans face upon returning home. Each concept and strategy discussed is akin to a tool in a hiker's pack, which is essential for the journey through the unpredictable terrain of post-war recovery.

In the hands of loved ones, these tools become the means to build a bridge over the chasms that trauma can create. Just as a bridge relies on its foundational supports, the success of psychedelic-assisted psychotherapy leans heavily on the strength of the relationships that gird a veteran. It is within the familial forge that the potency of these therapies is tempered and tested.

By adopting a stance of informed empathy and engaged support, family and friends can transform the recovery path into a shared expedition. This is not a passive engagement, akin to sitting beside a campfire, but rather an active partnership, resembling the shared labor of canoeing upstream. The companions of veterans are not mere spectators to the therapeutic process; they are co-navigators assisting in steering through the emotional currents.

In this shared journey, the roles of supporters evolve. They become co-healers facilitating the veteran's psychological rebirth through their growth and understanding. Think of a garden where both the gardener and the plants are nourished by caring; nurturing another life enriches one's own. This is the metamorphosis we envision—where assisting another becomes a conduit for one's transformation.

Let's recognize this chapter as an invitation to embark on a transformation journey. Psychedelic-assisted psychotherapy is a frontier of the mind and spirit, offering new vistas of healing and understanding. It asks supporters to be bold, vulnerable, and participate in a process that promises recovery and renewal.

CHAPTER 19

Addressing Feelings and Expectations

As family and friends of combat veterans, you embark on a shared journey that requires as much courage and preparation as the service members once summoned. The quest for healing through psychedelic-assisted psychotherapy invites veterans and their loved ones into a space of transformation. It's a path that demands vigilance in one's emotional landscape while navigating the unpredictable terrain of recovery and growth.

Self-care, for those who provide unwavering support to combat veterans embarking on a journey of psychedelic-assisted psychotherapy, is as critical as the guidance they offer. It is the art of maintaining one's inner calm and resilience amidst the emotional ebbs and flows that accompany the healing process of a loved one.

To be steadfast, like the keel of a ship, you must ensure that your emotional and psychological needs are met. This begins with the recognition of your own emotions as valid and important. It is natural to experience a spectrum of feelings—from hope to helplessness, from solidarity to isolation—as your veteran navigates their therapy. Acknowledge these emotions with compassion rather than judgment. Just as the keel moves with the water yet keeps the ship stable, allow your emotions to flow without letting them capsize your well-being.

Creating a self-care routine is akin to crafting a personalized map for your journey. This map should include activities that nourish your body, mind, and soul. Physical exercise, whether the solitary rhythm of a run or the collective energy of a team sport, can act as a catharsis, releasing the tension that builds up over time. Mental care might involve engaging in hobbies that require focus and creativity, like playing an instrument or building models, which can serve as a form of meditation, drawing your mind away from stress and anchoring you in the moment.

The psychological aspect of self-care often requires introspection. Journaling can be a private retreat, a space to voice your deepest concerns or celebrate small victories without fear of censure. Alternatively, counseling or therapy for yourself can be a sanctuary of verbalization, where a professional helps navigate the complex emotions that arise from your unique situation.

Social support is another pillar of self-care. Lean on friends, family, or support groups who understand your situation. Like sharing stories around a campfire, sharing your experiences with others can provide warmth and light in darker times. Remember that seeking connection is not a burden shared but a burden eased.

Rest and relaxation are not indulgent. They are necessities. Allow yourself periods of restorative quiet, as peaceful as the stillness of a lake at dusk. In these moments, mindfulness or meditation can be a raft, keeping you afloat amidst the waves of uncertainty. Yoga and tai chi can similarly help maintain your physical and emotional balance.

Remember, as you tend to your veteran, your well-being and well-being are not separate endeavors but concurrent missions. Self-care is tuning your instrument in the orchestra of healing, ensuring you can play your part in harmony with the melody of recovery. Investing in your resilience makes you a caregiver and a vital part of the work.

Expectations, when intertwined with the psyche, have the potential to shape one's reality in profound ways. In the pursuit of healing through psychedelic-assisted psychotherapy, it's vital to approach expectations not as rigid forecasts but as fluid aspirations. This flexible stance is deeply resonant with Buddhist teachings on the nature of attachment and the suffering it can engender.

Buddhism eloquently speaks to the root of suffering: attachment, not only to material possessions but also to outcomes and ideals. To cling too tightly to expectations is to set oneself on a path of potential disillusionment, much like over-tensioning a string risks its integrity. Conversely, to hold expectations too loosely may lead to a lack of engagement or commitment, disrupting the melody of progress. It is, therefore, through the middle way, a path of balanced expectations, that one may find peace.

The journey of healing with psychedelics, much like the practice of mindfulness, invites participants to dwell in the present moment to embrace the full spectrum of experiences without the burden of clinging to what 'should be.' It encourages an acceptance of what is, an acknowledgment that the landscape of the mind, like the natural world, is subject to its seasons and cycles.

Breakthroughs, in this therapeutic context, may indeed feel like reaching the summit of a great peak, offering expansive views and a sense of accomplishment. Setbacks, however, are not failures but integral parts of the journey, offering their lessons and opportunities for growth. They are akin to the valleys that nestle between mountains: necessary traverses on the path to the next summit.

In cultivating a Buddhist perspective, one learns to view each moment as complete, recognizing the impermanence of all experiences. This wisdom teaches that attaching to any particular outcome can be a source of suffering, for it is the nature of life to change and evolve. Instead, by cultivating equanimity and compassion, family and friends can offer a steadfast presence that is neither swayed by the highs of progress nor the lows of challenge.

Thus, managing expectations in the context of psychedelic therapy is not merely a psychological exercise but a profound practice of spiritual and emotional balance. It is an invitation to dance with the rhythm of life, to feel the music of existence in all its tones and textures, and to support your loved ones with a heart that is open, present, and accepting of each note as it comes.

Professional support stands as a beacon, offering clarity when the waters of personal involvement become murky with emotional turbulence. Therapists and counselors, trained in the art of psychological navigation, offer a compass by which you can steer through your internal storms. They serve as the lighthouse keepers, guiding you back to shore when you've drifted too far into the sea of emotional overwhelm.

These professionals can provide tools and strategies to manage the stress and burden of supporting someone through the healing process. They are akin to skilled mechanics who help you keep the machinery of your well-being in optimal condition. With their help, you can learn techniques for emotional regulation, such as deep breathing exercises or cognitive-behavioral strategies, which act as anchors in tumultuous times.

Support groups, too, are invaluable in this journey. They are like the collective strength of a team of climbers, all tethered together, ensuring that if one slips, the others can provide support. In these groups, shared experiences resonate like the harmonious chords of a well-tuned guitar, creating a melody of mutual understanding and compassion.

These resources are your allies, your co-navigators in this expedition, and they ensure that you do not shoulder the weight alone. By engaging with these forms of professional support, you maintain your capacity to be a constant source of strength for your veteran. This commitment to your support system is not a detour from the path of caregiving but an essential segment of the journey, ensuring you reach the desired destination together.

In the journey of healing, the role of the caregiver is as pivotal as that of the healer. As we conclude this chapter, it's paramount to recognize that self-care for those supporting veterans in psychedelic-assisted psychotherapy is not an ancillary consideration but a foundational element. It is the bedrock upon which the therapeutic process is built, the nurturer of resilience, and the cultivator of patience.

Ensuring your well-being is akin to carefully tuning a complex machine, ensuring that every cog and wheel functions in harmony, contributing to the greater purpose of recovery. Your emotional and psychological health is the lens through which you will view and interact with your veteran's experiences, and it must be clear and focused.

Throughout this chapter, we've navigated the significance of managing expectations with wisdom borrowed from Eastern philosophies, engaging in restorative practices, and the critical role of professional support. These are the tools at your disposal, the instruments you will use to compose a melody of support and care.

Remember, your journey is shared with your loved one as you walk this path. Your strength bolsters their courage, your resilience fortifies their spirit, and your well-being illuminates their way. By committing to your self-care with the same enthusiasm you dedicate to supporting your veteran, you become the unwavering beacon that guides them through the darkest nights toward the dawn of healing.

PART VI

Legal and Ethical Considerations

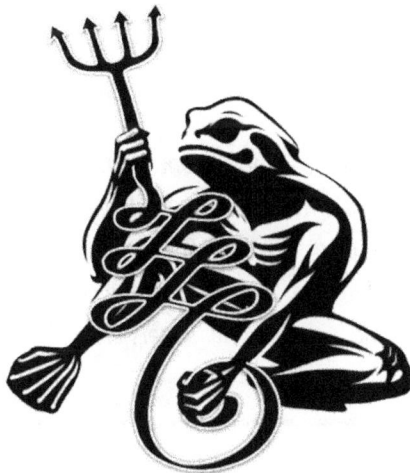

CHAPTER 20

The Legal Landscape

Disclaimer

The information presented in this chapter is provided for educational and informational purposes only and is not intended as legal advice. The legal status of psychedelic substances is complex and varies significantly across different jurisdictions. The laws governing the use, possession, distribution, and research of psychedelic substances are subject to frequent changes and can have profound implications.

Readers are urged to conduct their due diligence and consult with a qualified legal professional before making any decisions related to the therapeutic use of psychedelics. The individual is responsible for remaining abreast of current laws and regulations in their region or country.

The authors and publishers of this work do not advocate for or endorse the use of psychedelics where it is prohibited by law. Furthermore, while the therapeutic potentials of psychedelics are discussed, this should not be interpreted as medical advice. The path of medical treatment should always be undertaken with the support and supervision of a licensed healthcare provider.

The views expressed in this chapter are intended to foster understanding and dialogue regarding the legal landscape surrounding psychedelic substances. They should not be taken as an encouragement to partake in any illegal activities. The authors and publishers disclaim any liability for any direct or indirect repercussions arising from applying the information contained in this chapter.

The legal terrain of psychedelic substances is as varied and intricate as the psychological landscapes they are known to affect. Across the globe, governments and regulatory bodies are grappling with how to integrate the burgeoning evidence of the therapeutic benefits of psychedelics with existing drug policies steeped in decades of prohibition.

In the United States, the Controlled Substances Act (CSA) classifies psychedelics like psilocybin and LSD as Schedule I drugs, a category reserved for substances with a high potential for abuse and no accepted medical use. Despite this, the seismic shifts in public perception and scientific understanding create cracks in the once impenetrable legal bedrock.

Psilocybin: With its Schedule I classification, psilocybin is federally illegal to possess, use, or distribute. Yet, we are witnessing unprecedented decriminalization initiatives across the country. In Denver, Colorado, psilocybin was decriminalized in May 2019, followed by Oakland and Santa Cruz in California. Oregon went a step further, passing Measure 109 in November 2020, which legalized the regulated medical use of psilocybin. These local laws do not change federal policy but indicate a groundswell of support for therapeutic use, often led by veterans' advocacy groups that highlight the benefits of PTSD and other war-related traumas.

LSD: Despite its potential demonstrated in early psychiatric research and recent studies, LSD remains tightly controlled, with no legal distinction between its use for personal, medical, or research purposes under federal law. However, the interest in its therapeutic potential continues to grow, and discussions about rescheduling to acknowledge its medical value are gaining traction in scientific communities.

MDMA: Perhaps the most significant legal development in the psychedelic sphere is the FDA's designation of MDMA as a "breakthrough therapy" for PTSD. This status has expedited the review of clinical trial data, which could lead to rescheduling and medical legalization. MAPS' Phase III clinical trials represent the final stage needed for potential FDA approval, which could revolutionize the legal status of MDMA.

Ayahuasca: The legal narrative of Ayahuasca is rich with cultural, religious, and therapeutic landscapes. In the U.S., the Supreme Court has recognized the right of the União do Vegetal church to use Ayahuasca as a sacrament, setting a precedent for religious exemption. This legal recognition has not extended to therapeutic use outside of religious context, leaving a gray area for practitioners and patients alike.

Ibogaine: Ibogaine's status remains unchanged at the federal level, classified as a Schedule I substance. Yet, its potential for treating opiate addiction has prompted several cities to consider resolutions that would support medical research or decriminalize its use, signaling a shifting perspective on its value.

5-MeO-DMT: Similarly, 5-MeO-DMT is classified under Schedule I, but as research into its therapeutic benefits grows, especially for depression and anxiety, there is a possibility that its legal status could change to accommodate medical use.

The global perspective is similarly fragmented. Countries such as the Netherlands and Canada are adopting more progressive policies, allowing for specific legal uses of psychedelics. In contrast, nations like the U.K. and Australia maintain stringent controls, with ongoing debates about the potential for reform.

For veterans navigating this ever-changing legal realm, the implications are profound. Access to potentially life-altering therapies is not merely a matter of personal choice but of geographical and legal happenstance. The legal landscape of psychedelics is not static. Still, it is being reshaped by the winds of change—scientific advancements, advocacy, and a growing recognition of the therapeutic value of these substances.

The legal ramifications for unauthorized psychedelic use, possession, or distribution can be severe and life-altering. It is essential to understand that while the therapeutic and medicinal benefits of psychedelics are being studied and recognized in some regions, their legal status remains strictly controlled under the laws of many countries, particularly under international conventions like the United Nations Convention on Psychotropic Substances of 1971.

Federal and International Law:

Under federal law, particularly in the United States, most psychedelics are classified as Schedule I controlled substances. To be classified as Schedule I, substances are considered to have a high potential for abuse, no currently accepted medical use in treatment in the United States, And a lack of accepted safety for use under medical supervision. The ramifications of violating these regulations can include:

- *Criminal Charges*: Unauthorized possession, use, or distribution of psychedelics can lead to criminal charges, ranging from misdemeanors to felonies, depending on the quantity and intent (personal use vs. distribution).

- *Incarceration*: Convictions may result in jail or prison sentences, with the duration varying by state and federal law, as well as the amount of substance involved and prior criminal history.

- *Fines:* Substantial fines may be imposed, often in conjunction with or instead of incarceration.

- *Probation or Parole*: Individuals may be placed on probation or parole, requiring regular check-ins with a legal officer and compliance with specific terms, such as drug testing and employment.

- *Criminal Record:* Having a criminal record might affect future employment, educational opportunities, professional licensing, and eligibility for public assistance and housing.

- *Travel Restrictions:* A criminal record, especially for drug offenses, can restrict a person's ability to travel internationally.

State Laws

As mentioned, State laws may provide for sanctions that are either more lenient or more severe than federal laws. Some states have enacted measures to decriminalize or legalize the use of specific psychedelics, but these do not supersede federal law. Individuals in states with such laws still face potential federal charges.

- *Civil Penalties*: In some jurisdictions, civil penalties such as the forfeiture of property concerning the possession or distribution of illegal substances may also apply.

- *Employment and Professional Consequences*: The use of illegal substances can also have significant ramifications in a person's professional life, potentially leading to disciplinary action if such use violates professional conduct standards or employer policies.

- *Educational Consequences*: Students may face suspension or expulsion from educational institutions and loss of federal financial aid eligibility.

- *Impact on Active and Reserve Military*: For military personnel, the use of illegal substances can lead to discharge, loss of veterans' benefits, and other military justice consequences.

Individuals must be aware that despite the changing landscape of public opinion and scientific research regarding the therapeutic use of psychedelics, the legal system continues to impose strict penalties for activities that are not in compliance with the law. Even in therapeutic settings, the use of psychedelics must be authorized by and conducted under the supervision of licensed professionals and within the bounds of the regulatory framework.

This section underscores the high stakes involved in the use of psychedelics outside legal parameters and serves as a cautionary note about the breadth and depth of potential legal consequences. It is a stark reminder of the gap between emerging scientific understanding and existing legal structures.

The evolving legal discourse surrounding psychedelics reflects a broader societal shift toward a more empathetic understanding of mental health and the complexities of healing from trauma. As the boundaries of legality continue to be tested and expanded, those interested in psychedelic-assisted therapy must remain well-informed of their legal rights and the shifting sands of drug policy. This chapter guides through this dynamic and changing legal landscape, offering a beacon for those seeking healing in the face of legal uncertainties.

CHAPTER 21

Ethical Guidelines for Treatment

For veterans embarking on the path of psychedelic-assisted psychotherapy and their families standing in support, understanding the ethical landscape is as crucial as comprehending the treatment itself. This chapter is dedicated to illuminating the ethical standards that protect and empower you during this profound therapeutic journey.

Informed consent stands as the gateway to the journey of psychedelic-assisted psychotherapy. For veterans and their families, it is crucial to understand that this is more than a procedural formality; it is a comprehensive process that equips you with essential knowledge and prepares you for the path ahead. This journey of healing begins with a transparent conversation where you will learn about the potential benefits and the risks involved, the nature of the psychedelic experience, the course of treatment, and the aftercare considerations.

As a veteran or a supporting family member, you have the right to all this information presented in a manner that is accessible and easy to understand. This ensures you can make an informed and voluntary decision about whether to proceed with the treatment. It's a conversation that requires time and space, where questions are welcomed and encouraged. This process is about empowering you with confidence and clarity—ensuring that you do so with knowledge and assurance as you stand at the decision-making crossroads.

In the therapeutic sphere, especially when it intersects with the potent effects of psychedelics, your autonomy is of paramount importance. It is a foundational principle acknowledging your right to self-governance and to make decisions about your health and treatment. Therapists enter this space not as commanders but as allies, offering knowledge, support, and guidance while honoring your sovereign right to chart your course.

For families, this respect for autonomy involves supporting the veteran's decisions with trust and without judgment. It is about acknowledging the veteran's capacity for self-determination and understanding that, while the choices may be deeply personal, they warrant the same respect as any other medical or therapeutic decision. Through this mutual respect, the therapeutic journey maintains its integrity, ensuring that each step is with consent and agency.

Confidentiality: The sanctity of confidentiality in therapy forms the cornerstone of the therapeutic alliance. It is a solemn assurance that the intimate details of a veteran's experiences, thoughts, and feelings disclosed during therapy are held in strict confidence. This pledge of privacy is not merely a legal obligation but a moral one, reflecting the deep respect for the personal narratives entrusted to the therapist.

For veterans, confidentiality offers a secure space to unveil and explore the most guarded aspects of their inner lives without fear of judgment or exposure. It's an assurance that the stories of battle, the scars of service, and the tender moments of vulnerability will be shielded from the public eye, allowing for a candid and unencumbered exploration of the self.

As integral supporters in the healing journey, families play a pivotal role in honoring this confidentiality. Creating an environment where the veteran feels unreservedly safe to share within therapy is essential, knowing that these disclosures will not be discussed elsewhere without explicit consent. This extends beyond the therapy room and into the home, where conversations and information should be handled with discretion and empathy.

Confidentiality also encompasses the protection of records and communications. Strict professional standards bind therapists to prevent unauthorized access to therapy notes and session content. This includes ensuring that electronic communications, such as emails and messages, are securely managed in the digital age.

It is important to note that while confidentiality is a fundamental principle, there are exceptions where disclosure is legally mandated, such as when there is an immediate risk of harm to the veteran or others. These exceptions are outlined clearly in the informed consent process. They are in place to ensure the safety of all involved.

For veterans and their families, understanding the scope and limits of confidentiality builds trust in the therapeutic process. This trust allows for profound growth and healing, knowing that the space within which the therapeutic work occurs is both sacred and secure.

In the therapeutic setting, the imperative to maintain professional boundaries is paramount, mainly when dealing with the potent experiences that may arise during psychedelic-assisted psychotherapy. Understanding the ethical issues related to these boundaries, especially concerning dual relationships, is essential for veterans and their families.

A dual relationship occurs when a therapist has a secondary, significantly different relationship with their client—social, financial, or personal. These relationships can muddy the clear waters of the therapeutic dynamic, introducing risks of impaired judgment and the potential for exploitation or harm. For instance, if a therapist were also to be a veteran's business partner, friend, or romantic partner, their ability to remain objective and therapeutic could be compromised.

Dual relationships can blur the lines of professionalism. They can lead to a conflict of interests, where the veteran's needs might be unintentionally neglected in favor of the therapist's personal feelings or interests. This can result in a loss of trust, feelings of betrayal, or even harm to the veteran. Additionally, dual relationships can interfere with the therapist's ability to remain neutral, which is crucial for effective treatment.

A dual relationship can also exacerbate the power imbalance inherent in the therapeutic relationship. A veteran may feel unable to voice discomfort or terminate the therapy due to the additional connection, which can lead to ethical dilemmas and potential breaches of ethics.

Therapists must be vigilant in preventing such relationships from forming, as the ethics codes of most professional bodies strictly limit them due to the risks involved. Veterans and their families should be aware of the therapist's ethical obligations and feel empowered to discuss any concerns about potential dual relationships with the therapist.

If a dual relationship cannot be avoided—for example, in small or rural communities where social circles may overlap—the therapist must establish clear, written boundaries with the veteran, seek supervision, and take all necessary steps to protect the therapeutic integrity.

Veterans or family members who feel a dual relationship negatively impacts therapy can discuss their concerns with the therapist. The therapist is responsible for addressing these concerns and taking appropriate action, including referring the veteran to another provider.

Understanding the importance of professional boundaries and the problematic nature of dual relationships helps safeguard the therapeutic environment. It ensures that the focus remains on the veteran's healing journey, free from the complications arising from conflicting roles. This knowledge is crucial for families to support the veteran's therapeutic process and advocate for their best interests.

Transference is a psychological phenomenon when a person, in this case, a veteran, unconsciously redirects or projects feelings, desires, and expectations from past relationships onto the therapist. This can manifest in various ways, such as the veteran treating the therapist with the regard they might have shown a military superior, looking for a parental figure in the therapist, or even developing romantic feelings. Transference is not limited to positive emotions; it can also involve negative sentiments such as resentment or mistrust stemming from past experiences.

Countertransference is the therapist's emotional entanglement with the veteran. It's a reaction to the veteran's transference, where the therapist projects their background and issues onto the veteran. It can be excessive sympathy, irritation, or over-identification with the veteran's experiences.

Both transference and countertransference, if not recognized and appropriately managed, can lead to ethical complications. They can cloud clinical judgment, lead to boundary issues, and ultimately compromise treatment efficacy. For instance, a therapist may unknowingly encourage dependency in a veteran if the veteran's neediness gratifies them due to countertransference.

If left unchecked, these dynamics can disrupt the therapeutic alliance and may lead to adverse outcomes such as:

- Violation of boundaries, potentially resulting in inappropriate relationships.
- Misdiagnosis or mistreatment, as the therapist's countertransference, can bias their clinical perception.
- Harm to the veteran's emotional well-being if they feel misunderstood, rejected, or judged based on the therapist's projections.

Recognizing transference and countertransference involves a high level of self-awareness by the therapist and the veteran. Therapists must engage in regular self-reflection and seek supervision to remain objective. They may also educate the veteran about these phenomena as part of the therapy process, which can be therapeutic.

Veterans and their families should understand that while transference and countertransference can offer valuable insights into the veteran's inner world and the therapeutic relationship, they must be carefully navigated. It's beneficial for families to be aware of these dynamics as they can manifest in interactions outside therapy.

When transference or countertransference becomes disruptive, addressing it directly within the therapeutic relationship is crucial. This might involve the therapist discussing their observations of transference with the veteran to explore its origins and meanings. If countertransference is identified, the therapist may need to seek therapy or supervision to resolve personal issues affecting the treatment.

In cases where these dynamics severely hinder the therapy, it might be ethical for the therapist to refer the veteran to another provider. The primary goal is always the veteran's health and stability; sometimes, a new therapeutic relationship is the best way to ensure that.

Transference and countertransference are complex phenomena that, when managed well, can enrich the therapeutic process and lead to deeper self-understanding for the veteran. However, they require careful handling to avoid ethical breaches and protect the therapeutic environment's integrity. For veterans and their families, being informed about these issues is a decisive step in being proactive and participatory in therapy.

In the pursuit of healing, primarily through the avenue of psychedelic-assisted psychotherapy, the anchoring force is the reliance on evidence-based practices. These treatment modalities and therapeutic interventions have stood the test of rigorous scientific research and have been systematically evaluated in clinical settings to determine their effectiveness.

Evidence-based practices (EBPs) are therapies supported by peer-reviewed research and clinical studies. They are the gold standard in psychotherapy and involve methods proven to work through controlled experiments and clinical trials. EBPs are not static; they evolve as new research and data emerge, ensuring that the treatment approaches remain at the forefront of scientific knowledge.

For veterans and their families, the assurance that therapy is evidence-based is vital. It means that the interventions have been tested and shown to be beneficial for individuals with similar experiences and diagnoses. This level of validation can offer peace of mind that the chosen therapeutic path is innovative and has a foundation in proven outcomes.

Transparency is a key aspect of employing EBPs in therapy. Therapists should be open about their methods, including how they work, their aim, and what the current research says about their effectiveness. This openness allows veterans and their families to make informed decisions about engaging with therapeutic interventions.

Research in psychedelic-assisted psychotherapy is an ongoing endeavor. Clinical trials are conducted to understand the effects of psychedelics such as psilocybin, MDMA, and LSD on conditions commonly faced by veterans, such as PTSD, depression, and anxiety. The findings from these trials inform treatment protocols, ensuring that they are rooted in the most current scientific understanding.

Veterans and families need to critically evaluate the evidence supporting various treatment options. Not all treatments are suitable for everyone, and the efficacy of therapy can vary based on individual circumstances. It is appropriate to ask about the success rates of these treatments and whether they have been specifically tested among veteran populations.

Armed with evidence-based information, veterans and their families can make knowledgeable treatment decisions. Understanding the science behind the therapy enriches the therapeutic experience, fostering a collaborative environment where veterans and therapists work together toward healing.

Evidence-based practices in psychedelic-assisted psychotherapy are the map and compass for navigating the therapeutic journey—they inform where we are headed and the best paths to take. Veterans and their families are blessed to have mental health and medical and scientific communities that provide these innovative and scientifically validated treatments. This chapter guides understanding and engaging with these practices, providing a solid foundation for the therapeutic process and the journey toward healing.

Ethical considerations in psychedelic-assisted psychotherapy form a framework that safeguards the integrity of the treatment and the well-being of veterans. The scope of ethical issues in therapy is broad, encompassing various aspects of the therapeutic relationship and the standards of professional conduct that therapists are expected to uphold.

Ethical issues in therapy may arise in multiple contexts, including but not limited to managing confidential information, establishing and maintaining professional boundaries, handling transference and countertransference, and selecting and applying treatment modalities. Therapists are tasked with the complex duty of navigating these issues while prioritizing the care and respect of veterans.

Therapists are bound by a code of ethics established by professional regulatory bodies. This code serves as a beacon, guiding the therapeutic process. It ensures that therapists respect the rights and dignity of all clients, including veterans, who may have unique vulnerabilities due to their military experiences. The code typically covers principles such as non-maleficence, beneficence, autonomy, justice, and fidelity.

Informed consent goes beyond the initial treatment agreement; it is an ongoing dialogue. Veterans and their families have the right to be informed about the nature of the therapy, any risks involved, and the expected outcomes. Autonomy is respected by allowing veterans to make their own decisions regarding their treatment, free from coercion or undue influence.

Confidentiality breaches can be particularly damaging in the context of psychedelic-assisted psychotherapy due to the sensitive and some-times deeply personal nature of the experiences shared. Therapists must ensure that all communications and records are kept secure, and any discussion regarding the veteran's care with third parties must have explicit consent.

The principle of non-maleficence—avoiding harm—is especially per-tinent in psychedelic-assisted psychotherapy, given the powerful effects these substances can have on the mind and emotions. Therapists must be well-trained and knowledgeable about the potential risks associated with psychedelics and take all necessary precautions to mitigate them.

Inappropriate behavior, such as engaging in dual relationships, ex-ploiting the client-therapist relationship, or failing to provide the stan-dard of care, can have negative consequences. Therapists must always maintain a professional demeanor and work within the bounds of their competence.

Veterans and their families should feel empowered to address ethical concerns during therapy. Whether it's a question about the treatment approach, a potential confidentiality issue, or discomfort with a therapist's conduct, they should feel comfortable bringing these issues to the forefront. Therapists must foster an environment where open communication is welcomed and concerns are addressed promptly and effectively.

Veterans and their families have the right to seek further assistance if ethical issues are not satisfactorily resolved within the therapeutic context. This may involve contacting the therapist's professional board, a regulatory agency, or an independent ethics committee.

Ethical considerations are not mere formalities but integral to therapeutic work's fabric. This chapter aims to provide veterans and their families with a thorough understanding of the ethical landscape in psychedelic-assisted psychotherapy. By highlighting these issues and the mechanisms for addressing them, the goal is to ensure a treatment experience that is as ethically sound as it is transformative, where the veteran's welfare is the highest priority.

Veterans and their families should know that ethical concerns can be complex and multifaceted. If ethical issues arise, it is crucial to address them directly with the therapist or, if necessary, through the appropriate channels, such as licensing boards or professional ethics committees.

Understanding the boundaries and ethical considerations of the therapeutic relationship is crucial for veterans and their families. It fosters a treatment environment conducive to healing and growth, and it ensures that the focus remains firmly on the well-being and recovery of the veteran. Familiarity with these principles helps ensure that the journey through psychedelic-assisted psychotherapy is navigated with the utmost care and respect for the therapeutic process.

In psychedelic-assisted psychotherapy, the safety and welfare of veterans are of the utmost importance. Ensuring the well-being of those who have served our country extends beyond the bounds of traditional care into physical and psychological support during and after therapy sessions. This comprehensive approach to safety is critical in facilitating an effective and empathetic healing process.

Before embarking on therapy, a thorough medical screening is essential. This screening helps to identify any physical health conditions or medications that could interact with psychedelic substances. Veterans and families should expect a detailed review of medical history and possibly a physical examination as part of this preparation. Veterans must be forthcoming about their health to ensure their physical safety.

During psychedelic therapy sessions, close monitoring is key. The therapy team should be trained to respond to both the physical and emotional needs that may arise. This might include managing changes in blood pressure or heart rate, as well as providing reassurance or psychological support during intense moments of the psychedelic experience.

The presence of a trusted individual, whether a therapist or a family member, can provide immense comfort. Families can play a pivotal role by being present before and after sessions, offering emotional support, or simply being there to listen. This supportive presence can make all the difference in helping veterans feel secure and grounded.

The setting in which veterans return after therapy is just as important as the therapeutic setting itself. Families can help create a calm environment that promotes relaxation and reflection. This might involve preparing a quiet space, being available to talk, or ensuring the veteran has no immediate responsibilities that could add stress. Despite careful planning, challenging moments can occur. Responsive support means having a plan for managing complex emotional or psychological reactions. Therapists will guide how to navigate these moments, and families should feel prepared to assist in this supportive role.

The period following a psychedelic therapy session is critical for integration—the process of making sense of the experience and incorporating insights into daily life. Aftercare may include additional therapy sessions, support groups, or wellness activities. Families can encourage participation in these resources and offer a listening ear as veterans articulate their experiences.

In the unlikely event of a medical or psychological emergency, clear protocols should be in place. Veterans and families should be informed about these protocols, how to recognize an emergency, and whom to contact. This preparedness is a vital part of ensuring safety.

The safety and welfare of veterans in psychedelic-assisted psychotherapy hinge on meticulous preparation, vigilant monitoring, and a supportive network. This chapter provides veterans and their families with an understanding of the comprehensive measures taken to protect their well-being throughout the therapeutic process, ensuring that the journey toward healing is pursued with the highest regard for safety.

When seeking a therapist for psychedelic-assisted psychotherapy, veterans and their families must ensure that the practitioner is not only credentialed but also possesses a deep and nuanced understanding of the specific demands of this form of therapy. It is essential to have comprehensive knowledge of what constitutes professional competence in this specialized field, from educational background and licensure to years of practice and specialized training. We will discuss this topic in depth in the next chapter.

Accountability is a fundamental pillar in the ethical practice of psychedelic-assisted psychotherapy. Therapists are ethically obliged to provide the highest quality of care, which encompasses adhering to meticulously established protocols, engaging in best practices, and maintaining a commitment to professional development.

Ethical guidelines dictate that therapists must follow evidence-based protocols specifically designed for psychedelic therapy. This ensures that care is administered safely, respectfully, and effectively, minimizing risks and optimizing therapeutic outcomes. These protocols are not static; they evolve with ongoing research and clinical insights, requiring therapists to stay informed and integrate new findings into their practice.

The therapeutic process is, by nature, collaborative. Veterans and their families are encouraged to provide feedback on their care, an essential component of clinical governance.

Ethically, therapists must welcome and value this feedback, seeing it as an opportunity for continual improvement rather than criticism.

Veterans and their families have the right to expect care that is not only competent but also compassionate, culturally sensitive, and personalized. Therapists must respect each veteran's unique needs and values, providing care aligned with the individual's goals and life context.

It is a veteran's right and an aspect of the therapeutic alliance to voice concerns if the care provided falls short of ethical or professional standards. Ethical practice involves creating an environment where veterans and their families can express concerns without fear of retribution or dismissal.

When issues are raised, therapists have a responsibility to address them promptly and effectively. Suppose a concern points to a gap in the therapist's knowledge or skill. In that case, ethical guidelines require them to seek additional supervision, training, or consultation to rectify this gap.

The ethical framework within psychedelic-assisted psychotherapy places a high value on accountability in care. This framework ensures that veterans receive effective treatment with the utmost ethical consideration. For veterans and their families, understanding this aspect of care provides a foundation for engaging with therapy in a way that is empowered, informed, and secure in the knowledge that the therapist is held to the highest ethical standards.

The emergent field of psychedelic-assisted psychotherapy, like any innovative domain, is replete with complexities and unknowns. Ethical practice within this space is defined by a commitment to professional integrity, continuous education, and the flexibility to adapt to new challenges and information.

Ethical guidelines mandate that therapists commit to lifelong learning to enhance their understanding and stay current with the latest developments in psychedelic research and therapeutic techniques. This commitment ensures they can provide the most informed and effective care possible.

Therapists must actively seek consultation and supervision, especially when faced with clinical uncertainties or novel situations that fall outside their current expertise. This is a key aspect of ethical practice, allowing for peer review and sharing knowledge within the professional community to serve clients better.

Ethics in psychedelic therapy also require flexibility and responsiveness. Therapists should be prepared to modify treatment approaches as new evidence emerges and as they learn more about each veteran's unique response to therapy.

Veterans and their families are integral to the therapeutic process. Ethically, therapists should involve them in discussions about the treatment approach, especially when navigating the less charted aspects of psychedelic therapy. This collaborative approach respects the veteran's autonomy. It recognizes the valuable insights families can provide based on their intimate knowledge of the veteran's experiences and needs.

The therapeutic journey is one of mutual growth. Veterans and their families should be encouraged to engage in the learning process, understanding that the field is evolving and that their feedback and experiences contribute to the collective knowledge base of psychedelic therapy.

Ethical practice in the context of psychedelic-assisted psychotherapy involves a constellation of principles: a dedication to ongoing education, the humility to seek guidance, the flexibility to adapt, and the recognition of the veteran and family as co-navigators in the journey. It's about forging a path through uncertainties with a compass set on ethical integrity and a continually redrawn map with the insights of collective experience and scientific progress.

As we conclude this chapter, we reaffirm our commitment to illuminating the ethical framework that serves as both the foundation and the guiding light for psychedelic-assisted psychotherapy. Though ripe with potential for profound healing, this journey is navigated within a structure that ensures the highest standards of safety, integrity, and respect for the dignity of all veterans and their families.

We have explored the essential elements that constitute the bedrock of ethical practice in this emerging field—from informed consent to cultural sensitivity, from the rigorous training and competence of therapists to their accountability in care. Each element is a piece in the intricate puzzle of psychedelic therapy, placed together to create a picture of therapeutic excellence.

Informed consent is an important procedural checkpoint. It serves as the start of a partnership based on transparency and trust. It is your right as veterans and families to be fully informed about what psychedelic therapy entails, the potential risks and benefits, and to have your autonomy respected at every turn.

Understanding the significance of licensure and the continuous professional development of therapists empowers you to seek out those who are qualified and dedicated to maintaining their clinical acumen. The specialized training in psychedelic therapy that your therapists have undertaken is assurance that they can competently guide you through these experiences with skill and sensitivity.

We acknowledge therapists' and coaches' unique roles, emphasizing that while both can be instrumental in your journey, they serve different purposes and are bound by different ethical guidelines.

Navigating uncertainties with adaptability and a commitment to learning reflects the evolving nature of this field. It is a shared journey where the expertise of the therapist and the lived experiences of veterans and families coalesce to forge a therapeutic alliance that is robust, dynamic, and transformative.

Finally, this chapter speaks to the profound respect we hold for the sacrifices made by veterans. It is crafted to be a guide that offers clarity and confidence as you, the veterans, and your families consider or engage in psychedelic-assisted psychotherapy. It is designed to ensure that your therapeutic experience is effective and ethically grounded, honoring your service and the vital role of your families in the healing process.

Finding Professionals

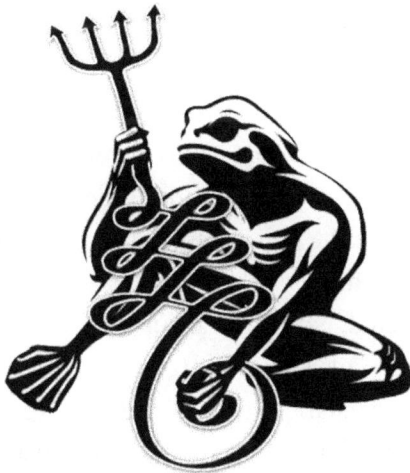

CHAPTER 22

Finding the Right
Professional Guide

When seeking a therapist for psychedelic-assisted psychotherapy, veterans and their families must ensure that the therapist possesses knowledge, experience, and a deep and nuanced understanding of the specific demands of this form of therapy. It is essential to have comprehensive understanding of what constitutes professional competence in this specialized field, from educational background and licensure to years of practice and specialized training. With so many therapists to choose from, how does one pick? There is a guide, albeit not the Rosetta Stone, but a simple, practical guide to help in your search.

At the heart of any therapeutic process lies the therapeutic alliance, the collaborative and empathetic bond between therapist and client, which is a cornerstone of successful outcomes, particularly in the nuanced field of psychedelic therapy. This is not a one-size-fits-all alliance. It is based on mutual respect, trust, and understanding. It is tailored to the individual needs of the person embarking on the journey.

The question of whether a therapist's sex or gender aligns with that of the veteran is layered, with clinical guidelines offering no prescriptive path. The advantages of a same-sex/gender therapist might include a perceived shared understanding of specific life experiences, potentially fostering a quicker rapport. However, therapy can also benefit from the diversity of perspectives that a therapist of a different sex/gender can provide, challenging veterans to confront various aspects of their psyche in a safe and therapeutic setting. The decision here is deeply personal and varies from one individual to another, reflecting each veteran's comfort level and personal history.

Fondness for a therapist is not a prerequisite for progress. However, liking your therapist can be an integral part of the therapeutic alliance, often leading to a stronger connection and greater willingness to engage in the therapeutic process. It is crucial, however, to discern between personal liking and professional respect, the latter being more significant for a therapy based on trust and expertise.

Choosing the right therapist extends beyond credentials; it is about character and attributes. A suitable therapist for psychedelic therapy should possess not only a profound understanding of the veteran's unique experiences but also the empathy to connect with them on a human level. They must be a skilled navigator capable of guiding the veteran through the intricate layers of their consciousness. They must exhibit patience, a non-judgmental stance, cultural competence, and a solid ethical grounding. Above all, they must provide a safe harbor for veterans to explore and integrate their experiences without fear of being overwhelmed by the tides of their psyche.

In the end, selecting a therapist is akin to choosing a fellow mountaineer for an arduous climb; one looks for experience, sure-footedness, and the ability to maintain composure in the face of the unexpected. The relationship is a partnership, with both parties invested in healing and growth. As we venture into the realm of psychedelic therapy, where the landscapes of mind and emotion are as vast and complex as any mountain range, the therapeutic alliance stands as our base camp, essential for any successful expedition.

Educational and Credential Requirements

For those who have bravely served and their families who are seeking guidance through psychedelic-assisted psychotherapy, the educational and credential requirements of a therapist are a testament to their proficiency and commitment to ethical practice. A robust educational background is crucial, as it underpins the therapist's understanding of complex psychological theories and therapeutic methodologies.

While the traditional paths of clinical psychology, psychiatry, social work, mental health counseling, and marriage and family therapy remain foundational, the field of psychedelic therapy often draws from a broader spectrum of psychological disciplines. Degrees accredited by bodies like the APA, NASW, ACA, or AAMFT ensure that therapists have met standardized benchmarks of academic rigor and professional training to meet the rigors of national licensure standards.

Beyond these core pathways, institutions such as Naropa University and the California Institute of Integral Studies (CIIS) offer specialized programs in depth psychology and transpersonal psychology. These disciplines delve into the deeper realms of the psyche. They are well-suited to the transformative nature of psychedelic therapy. They emphasize a holistic approach to mental health that aligns closely with the philosophies underlying many psychedelic therapies.

Depth psychology explores the unconscious aspects of the psyche and is particularly relevant to psychedelic therapy. It can bring unconscious material to the surface. Therapists with a background in depth psychology are trained to navigate these deep psychological waters, making them well-equipped to guide patients through the profound experiences often encountered with psychedelic substances.

Transpersonal psychology extends beyond the individual to consider broader aspects of the human experience, including spirituality and consciousness. Given that psychedelic experiences can entail transcendent or spiritual dimensions, therapists trained in transpersonal psychology can be particularly adept at facilitating and integrating these experiences.

Regardless of the educational path, accreditation from a recognized body is critical. It assures a level of academic quality and ethical standards. Additionally, state licensing boards provide further oversight, ensuring that therapists are educated and continually held to current professional and ethical standards.

Licensure and Continuous Learning

Licensure is the keystone in a therapist's professional journey, formally recognizing their competence and readiness to provide quality mental healthcare. For veterans and their families seeking psychedelic-assisted psychotherapy, understanding the nuances of licensure is vital to ensuring that the therapist they choose is qualified and has met all the rigorous standards required to practice.

Achieving licensure is a demanding process that builds upon the master's level educational foundation a therapist has laid. It requires a commitment to at least two years of full-time work, translating to around 40 hours per week, during which the therapist garners practical experience. This period is an intensive time of growth, where theoretical knowledge is applied in real-world scenarios under the supervision of experienced professionals.

The postgraduate journey includes a minimum of a hundred hours of direct supervised clinical work, where therapists refine their skills and learn to navigate the complexities of client care under the tutelage of a licensed supervisory clinician. This supervision is a critical phase, providing fledgling therapists with mentorship and the opportunity to discuss cases, receive feedback, and develop their clinical judgment.

Beyond initial training, therapists must engage in ongoing education, accumulating hundreds of hours in continuing education units (CEUs). These educational activities ensure that therapists stay current with the latest research findings, therapeutic techniques, and best practices in the field, including those related to psychedelic therapy.

The final hurdle in the licensure process is a rigorous, nationally sanctioned licensure examination. This comprehensive test assesses a therapist's readiness to practice independently, ensuring they have mastered a broad range of knowledge and skills necessary for effective therapeutic practice.

For veterans and their families, the therapist's licensure guarantees professional accountability. It indicates that the therapist has completed advanced education, honed their skills in a supervised setting, and is committed to ongoing professional development. It is evidence of their dedication to meeting the highest standards of their profession.

When selecting a therapist, veterans and their families should be encouraged to inquire about their professional licensure status. A therapist's willingness to discuss their licensure journey can indicate transparency and a commitment to ethical practice.

The licensure process is designed to protect the public and ensure that those providing psychotherapy services are competent at delivering care safely and effectively. For those embarking on the journey of psychedelic-assisted psychotherapy, the licensure of a therapist is a critical factor to consider, assuring that the therapist is equipped to guide veterans through the transformative process with skill, integrity, and a commitment to lifelong learning.

Now, let's address the role of a 'Coach." Both coaches and therapists play significant roles, yet their functions, training, and the scope of their work differ markedly. Understanding these differences is crucial for veterans and their families as they navigate the options for support and care.

A coach is often focused on goal-setting, personal growth, and development. They work with clients to identify objectives, develop strategies to achieve them, and foster accountability.

Coaching does not typically involve diagnosing or treating mental health disorders. Instead, it is action-oriented, concentrating on the present and future rather than delving into past experiences.

Coaches may come from various backgrounds and do not require the same level of credentialing as licensed therapists. While coaching certifications are available through organizations like the International Coach Federation (ICF), they do not equate to the state-regulated licensure that therapists must obtain. Coaches are not typically required to complete postgraduate supervised clinical work or comprehensive licensing exams.

Coaches cannot provide psychotherapy unless they are also trained and licensed as therapists. Their work is generally educational and developmental, improving performance, relationships, and life satisfaction. Coaches are not legally allowed to diagnose or treat mental health conditions, and their services are not a substitute for psychotherapy when such intervention is needed.

A coach must recognize their competence's boundaries and avoid engaging in therapeutic interventions. They should be transparent with clients about the limits of their role and practice within the ethical guidelines of their coaching certification.

While coaches may offer support for personal development and goal clarity, they are not equipped to handle the psychological complexities that can arise from psychedelic experiences. Without the clinical training to navigate such deep psychological processes, coaches should not guide clients through psychedelic experiences or the integration process that follows.

There may be instances where a coach and therapist work collaboratively to support a client. For example, a veteran might see a therapist for mental health concerns while working with a coach on life goals and personal development. In such cases, clear communication and defined roles are essential to ensure the veteran's needs are met without overlap or conflict between the services provided.

For veterans and their families considering support services, it's essential to differentiate between the roles of a coach and a therapist. While a coach can be a valuable resource for motivation, goal-setting, and personal growth, they do not replace the expertise and clinical skills of a licensed therapist, especially in contexts involving mental health and the profound experiences associated with psychedelic-assisted psychotherapy. When selecting a professional for support, matching the individual's needs with the appropriate provider is important, whether for therapeutic healing or coaching toward personal aspirations.

Specialized Training in Psychedelic Therapy

Psychedelic therapy for combat veterans demands more than just a foundational understanding of psychotherapy—it requires a profound immersion into specialized paradigms that cater to the unique psychological and emotional landscapes of veterans. The evolving domain of psychedelic therapy is characterized by two dominant training models: harm reduction and psychedelic-assisted psychotherapy. While the former provides strategies for those already exploring psychedelics, the latter offers a comprehensive framework that supports the entire journey, including the preparation, the ceremonial experience, and the post-experience integration.

Institutions like the Integrative Psychiatry Institute, MAPS, and CIIS provide immersive programs that last several months to a year, ensuring that therapists are trained and further transformed through the knowledge and experience they gain. These programs offer an extensive toolkit designed to navigate the complexities of psychedelic therapy, integrating interdisciplinary perspectives from psychology, medicine, spirituality, and philosophy.

A therapist trained in the harm reduction model might offer guidance to veterans who are already self-exploring psychedelics, seeking to understand and integrate these experiences into their daily lives. However, for a structured and ceremonial therapeutic experience, therapists with extensive training in psychedelic-assisted psychotherapy are indispensable. These therapists undergo rigorous programs that prepare them to guide veterans through the nuanced process of preparation, the profound experience of the psychedelic journey, and the critical phase of integration, where insights are infused into the veteran's life.

When seeking a therapist for psychedelic-assisted therapy, it is imperative to look beyond mere certificates. The story behind a therapist's training—their program's length, depth, and content—reveals much about their capacity to navigate this delicate terrain. A weekend certificate may hint at an interest. Still, it is the long-term, committed relationship with psychedelic studies that forges a therapist capable of steering veterans through psychedelic therapy.

Understanding the distinction between these training models is as crucial as knowing the difference between a life jacket and a ship when setting sail on the tumultuous seas of the mind. Veterans and their families must arm themselves with knowledge, ask pointed questions, and choose their therapeutic captain with wisdom. In this transformative voyage, the therapist's qualifications and training differentiate a perilous drift from a life-altering journey across the inner landscape.

Years of practice enrich a therapist's skillset, providing them with a broad spectrum of case studies and the sensibility to navigate complex emotional landscapes. However, the freshness and adaptability of newer therapists, often trained in the latest research and methodologies, are also valuable. A blend of experience and new perspectives can be ideal in a therapeutic setting, offering a balance of tried-and-tested approaches with innovative strategies.

As this chapter draws to a close, we anchor in the recognition that the journey of psychedelic therapy for combat veterans is a sacred and complex passage that requires a navigator of the highest caliber. Specialized training paradigms of harm reduction and psychedelic-assisted psychotherapy are more than educational paths. They facilitate the alchemical transformation of therapists into healers who can proficiently guide veterans through the rugged terrain of their psyche.

The path of such a therapist is not measured by the passage of weekends but by the transformative months or years spent in rigorous study and practice. Therapists are endowed with a diverse and rich toolkit through institutions like the Integrative Psychiatry Institute, MAPS, and CIIS, harmonizing the wisdom of psychology, medicine, spirituality, and philosophy. This toolkit is not for mere intervention but for crafting a rite of passage that honors the full spectrum of the veteran's experience.

In the search for a guide in this profound journey, veterans and their families are called to look deep into the heart of a therapist's qualifications. A certificate is but a map; it is the depth of training and the breadth of understanding that chart the course. For those who have served in combat, this therapeutic voyage can be a beacon back to life, a passage from the shadow of war into the light of peace.

As we conclude, let us hold fast to the knowledge that the therapist's expertise is the vessel that carries the veteran through the storm. In the solemnity of this journey, the right therapist does not merely buoy the spirit but sets the sails for new horizons. This voyage is about navigating the inner cosmos and returning enriched and transformed, ready to plant one's feet firmly on the ground of a new beginning. The journey is deep, the work is profound, and the potential for healing and wholeness is as vast as the mind's uncharted waters.

VIII

Concluding Chapters

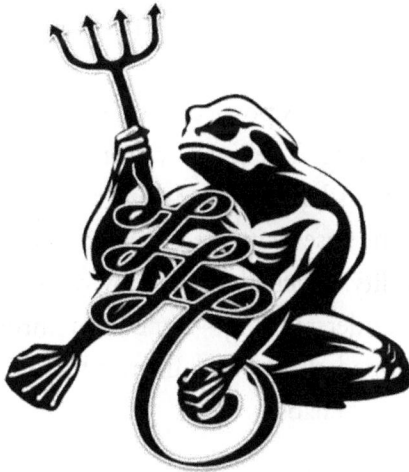

CHAPTER 23

Ascending Emergent Emotional Terrain

In the quest for peace that many combat veterans embark upon, the terrain of the mind can be as treacherous and unknown as any battlefield they have faced. The path does not end with the cessation of conflict; instead, it begins anew as they seek to understand the transformation of their emotional and psychological landscapes in the aftermath of war. This chapter is dedicated to the brave souls navigating these emergent emotional landscapes, illuminated by the beacon of psychedelic-assisted psychotherapy.

The Alchemy of Transformation: From Turmoil to Tranquility

The emotional upheavals post-conflict in the warrior's heart can be profound and perplexing. The journey from the cacophony of war to the possibility of inner silence is not merely a transition but an alchemical process, where the base elements of turmoil can be transmuted into the gold of tranquility. Psychedelic therapy offers a chalice brimming with the elixir of understanding—a medium through which understanding can be sipped slowly and from which serenity can emerge amidst the remnants of chaos.

We venture deeper into this metamorphosis, acknowledging the sage perspectives of Ken Wilber and Roger Walsh, luminaries who have charted the intricate maps of consciousness and transformation. With their insights as our guide, we recognize that each warrior's psyche is a microcosm of the universe, where battles fought are akin to the stars—numerous and distant, yet capable of illuminating the night sky of the mind.

The warrior in the throes of psychedelic therapy is not a mere by-stander in their journey of healing. They are the alchemist and the vessel, the philosopher and the stone, melding their will with ancient wisdom to forge a renewed self. As they ingest the sacraments of healing under the guidance of a skilled therapist, they encounter the multiplicity of their being. It is a plunge into the depths of the psyche, where the turbulence of war's memories can be transformed into pillars of strength and understanding.

In this sacred space, the *Warriors of the Mind* confront their shadows not with weapons but with the light of awareness. Psychedelics serve as a catalyst, an agent provoking the profound inner shifts necessary for metamorphosis. They beckon the subconscious to the forefront, inviting it to dialogue with the conscious mind. Here, in the liminal space of transformation, the soldiers' experiences are reframed, their traumas acknowledged, and their identities reconstituted.

The process is neither swift nor easy. It resembles the laborious turning of the alchemist's wheel, rotating with intention and care. Each cycle brings the warrior closer to the heart of their turmoil, allowing them to understand its composition and, ultimately, to recast it in the light of their evolving consciousness.

The transformation is a path of change, with each turn a narrative of struggle, resilience, and rebirth. The insights gained from such journeys are not merely personal victories but collective treasures, adding to the repository of human experience and wisdom. In this shared vault of knowledge, the lessons of Wilber and Walsh serve as invaluable gems, enlightening the paths of those who tread the road from turmoil to tranquility.

This alchemy of the soul is the central rite of passage for the returning warrior. It is a sacred art, a mystical science that demands as much faith as it does bravery. Through the vessel of psychedelic therapy, warriors are offered the potential to transmute the leaden weight of their past into the golden promise of a tranquil future. It is a future where the armor can be laid down, and the heart can beat not in the rhythm of war but in the peaceful cadences of a life reclaimed.

The Spiral Dynamics of the Psyche

The pilgrimage of the post-combat psyche is a deeply personal and singular journey, like a fingerprint that bears unique identifiers of one's experiences. It is a reminder of the complexity of the human condition that no two paths of healing are identical, each shaped by the distinct contours of an individual's encounters, both in war and in the aftermath of peace. Aside from Abraham Maslow's Hierarchy of Needs, the theory of Spiral Dynamics, a nuanced model of human development and consciousness, provides rich frameworks for understanding these varied pathways.

While Maslow highlights the simplicity of a linear progression, Spiral Dynamics suggests that development follows a dynamic, spiraling path where each turn represents an evolution of understanding and a reorientation of one's perspective on the self, society, and the broader cosmos. Hand in hand, these theories can be a guide to understanding what happens after a psychedelic journey.

In the intricacies of human evolution and psychological growth, Spiral Dynamics and Maslow's Hierarchy of Needs are compelling choreographers, guiding us through the ascending spirals of our unfolding consciousness. The dance begins in the realm of the archaic— raw, survivalist, and instinctual behaviors that form the bedrock of our being, much like the base of Maslow's famed pyramid where physiological needs demand immediate attention.

From this primal foundation, the spiral ascends, unfurling through ever more complex and nuanced levels of existence. We journey through the landscape of our animalistic and security needs, where the primal impulses of survival still whisper but are tempered by a burgeoning awareness of safety and the desire for order. This echoes the second tier of Maslow's structure, where once the basic needs for food and shelter are met, our gaze turns toward the security that allows us to sleep soundly and plan for tomorrow.

The spiral then twists upward through the realm of power and impulsivity, capturing the raw energy and drive that compels us to leave our mark on the world. It's a stage of ego and conquest, where we test our limits and assert our will. Parallel to this is Maslow's stage of love and belonging, where our social instincts flourish, and we seek connection and acceptance from our peers.

Ascending further, the spiral winds through the domain of order and rules, reflecting a yearning for structure and understanding. It is a stage where the chaos of raw impulses gives way to the dance of society's rhythms, orchestrated by laws and norms. In Maslow's hierarchy, this phase correlates with the realm of esteem, where recognition and respect become the melody we chase, and our achievements become the notes that define our song.

Reaching toward the skies, the spiral elevates us to the levels of achievement and success, paralleling Maslow's realm of self-esteem. Here, pursuing personal goals and validating accomplishments become the fuel that propels us further along our upward trajectory.

But the journey does not end with personal triumph. The spiral extends into ecological awareness and relational harmony, where understanding our interconnectedness with all life and the planet becomes paramount. Here, our narrative expands to include not just the self but the collective, mirroring the more elusive stage of Maslow's model—self-actualization, where the fulfillment of potential and the realization of one's true self take center stage.

The spiral then reaches toward the integrative, systematic, and synergetic realms, where the complexities of existence are embraced, and a systemic view of life is adopted. Here, we start to perceive the intricate connections that form the framework of life, creating a complex and harmonious image. At the zenith of the spiral lies the holistic, universal, and global vision—the final level, where the boundaries between the self and the universe blur, and a universal consciousness emerges. This ultimate stage of Spiral Dynamics aligns with the pinnacle of Maslow's pyramid, transcending self-actualization and venturing into the territory of self-transcendence. Here, the individual's journey becomes indistinguishable from the universal quest for meaning, belonging, and the ultimate truth.

Through the lens of these two models, we perceive the evolution of the self as a series of ascending spirals, where each level brings us closer to realizing our fullest potential, our most profound truths, and our deepest connections to the world and each other. This section of our narrative is a celebration of that ascent, an ode to the journey that each of us undertakes, from the archaic echoes of our beginnings to the universal song of our shared destiny.

As veterans embark on this journey of self-discovery, particularly under the influence of psychedelics, they engage with the pyramid and spiral in a profound dance of transformation. The psychedelics act as a catalyst, often accelerating the journey through different levels of being and consciousness, offering new vantages from which to view their internal and external worlds. Each level delineates a pattern of thinking and being that is more complex, integrative, and encompassing than the last.

In the spiraling journey of the combat veteran's psyche, the first turns are often shadowed by the primal instincts of survival—the very base of Maslow's pyramid where physiological and safety needs are the most pressing. Here, amid the echoes of war's dissonance, the veteran grapples with the foundational needs of security and community, seeking to reestablish a sense of stability that conflict has disrupted. These initial stages resonate deeply with the warrior's experience, where the instinct to protect and the longing to belong wage a silent war within.

As the veteran ascends through the spiral, their quest mirrors the upward movement through Maslow's levels of needs. The spiral's turn toward power, autonomy, and order reflects the veteran's struggle with self-esteem and the drive for mastery and recognition. Here, the warrior ethos, emphasizing strength and leadership, meets the internal conflicts that arise in the aftermath of war. Psychedelic therapy can serve as a gentle guide through these waves, softening the rigid structures of a militarized mindset and ushering the soul into the higher, more fluid states of being where achievements and accolades give way to the search for meaning and self-realization.

Further, along the spiral, the veteran encounters realms where the need for community and connection unfolds—a stage that echoes Maslow's social needs. It is a space where the veteran can begin to reconcile the solitary identity of the warrior with the interconnectedness of their civilian life, finding common ground and shared purpose with those around them.

At the higher turns of the spiral, the veteran reaches the stages of integration and wholeness, where the polarities of self and other, war and peace, start to blur and merge. This phase of the journey is akin to Maslow's self-actualization stage, where personal potential begins to flower, and the sense of being part of something larger becomes clear. Here, under the influence of psychedelics, profound epiphanies may occur, offering the veteran glimpses of an individual reality deeply connected to the web of life.

Navigating the spiral is a dance with light and shadow, an intricate choreography of progress and occasional regression. Psychedelic experiences, while potent and revelatory, can also unveil the abysses within the psyche that demand careful, compassionate integration. The principles of Spiral Dynamics serve as a map through this complex terrain, offering both veteran and therapist insight into the stages of growth and the challenges they may bring.

In this expansive view, the spiral is a metaphor—a living method for growth, a dynamic blueprint for the veteran's healing path. With each loop through the spiral, aided by the catalytic power of psychedelics, the veteran discovers new insights and faces fresh challenges, each contributing to the construction of a more nuanced and harmonious self.

The ascent through the Spiral Dynamics of the Psyche intertwined with the levels of Maslow's hierarchy is an enduring invitation to change, grow, and become. It is a recognition that the journey of self-discovery and healing does not end with the cessation of conflict but continues, spiraling upward toward new vistas of understanding and states of being, where the ultimate horizon is not a destination but a continual process of becoming.

In the profound journey of spiritual and personal evolution, each individual stands alone at the base of an immense monolith that reaches toward the heavens. This monolith embodies their life's trials, triumphs, and the transformative quest that lies ahead. It is a solo free climb, with no lead or follower, no safety of a belay. Each handhold and foothold represent the unique choices and challenges that must be navigated independently.

This lone quest of inner evolution is akin to ascending the spiral of consciousness and traversing the levels of Maslow's pyramid, where the path of growth is deeply personal. Here, one cannot be carried, nor can they carry another, for the weight of two climbers on a rope meant for one will only hinder the ascent. Each soul must engage with the climb at their own pace, discovering their rhythm, confronting their fears, and finding solace in their solitude.

The climb through the spiral and the pyramid is not a journey of companionship but of individual endeavor. To attempt to pull another up through the layers of transformation is to disrupt one's progress and to impose upon the other a pace and path that is not their own. The ascent requires self-reliance and the freedom to explore the personal depths and peaks that define the contours of one's soul.

Let your journey stand as a powerful example of personal transformation. Let it be a model that does not coerce but inspires, scaffolding others upward through the power of example. As you navigate the intricate twists of your path, be mindful that your ascent may serve as a beacon, casting light on the possibility of reaching greater heights. Be the silent influence that ignites a spark of motivation in others so they may see in your climb the potential for their own.

In this sacred and solitary expedition, each climber is the architect and the witness of their metamorphosis. Your evolution, marked by every moment of introspection and revelation, resonates with the cadence of your journey. While singular, it is a complexity of endless echoes in the expanse, inspiring others to listen.

As you ascend on your solitary climb, remember that the greatest gift you can offer is not to pull others along but to illuminate the path with the light of your growth. Let your journey be a clarion call that awakens the dormant climbers in their valleys, encouraging them to embark upon their ascent, to discover their strength, and to scale their spirals and pyramids in their own time, in their own way.

As the veteran ascends their monolith, encountering the silence of their solo climb, they are frequently graced with profound experiences that elude the grasp of conventional language— the ineffable encounters with the sublime, moments so saturated with meaning and mystery that they seem to exist in a realm beyond words. Psychedelic therapy often serves as the vessel to these uncharted waters, guiding the veteran to confront and reconcile with experiences of death and rebirth and sensations of unity with the cosmos that are as transformative as they are elusive.

In this sacred space of transformation, veterans may find themselves face to face with the most ancient of human quests—the search for meaning amid the mysterious. It is a quest undertaken by philosophers, theologians, and mystics throughout the ages. It is a journey across the continuum of human experience that connects the individual's quest to a universal narrative.

Within the folds of this chapter, we endeavor to illuminate the shadowed corners of these profound experiences. Drawing from the deep wells of Eastern and Western philosophy, we seek to contextualize the ineffable within the depths of human thought. The philosophies of the East, with their emphasis on the cyclical nature of life and the intricate dance of creation and destruction, offer a framework within which the experiences of death and rebirth can be understood as fundamental to the evolution of the self.

Western philosophy, with its roots in the exploration of being and existence, provides a lens through which the veteran's newfound sense of oneness with the cosmos can be viewed not as an anomaly but as an integral part of the human condition. Theology enters this dialogue with its rich history of interpreting mystical experiences, offering narratives that help frame these psychedelic journeys in the context of the soul's relationship with the divine.

Mythology, too, plays a vital role in resolving the ineffable. The mythic stories passed down through generations serve as a symbolic language that can encapsulate the profound and often paradoxical nature of psychedelic experiences. These stories and archetypes offer a way to communicate the transformative encounters that defy rational explanation, providing a shared vocabulary for deeply personal experiences yet universally resonant.

Empirical studies and expert opinions bridge these ancient wisdom traditions and contemporary understanding. The latest research in psychology and neuroscience offers insights into how psychedelics can rewire the brain, dissolving the barriers that compartmentalize our experiences and allowing for a holistic integration of the self. Experts in the field of psychedelic therapy provide practical strategies for veterans to reconcile these profound experiences, facilitating the integration of their visions and revelations into a coherent and meaningful worldview.

This quest to resolve the ineffable is not a pursuit of definitive answers but an exploration of possibilities. It invites the veteran to weave their narratives and find their symbols and meanings within the vast human experience. As we transition into the profound personal nature of transformation, we recognize that while the ineffable may be shared, its resolution is deeply personal. The veteran's journey through death and rebirth, through unity with the cosmos, is a solo voyage—a passage that each must navigate in their own time, with their compass, drawing their map of the world that the touch of the ineffable has irrevocably altered.

The Profound Personal Nature of Transformation

As we emerge from the enigmatic embrace of the ineffable, we enter the sanctum of personal transformation, a domain where the journey of change is as intimate and profound as the psyche that bears its imprints. This metamorphosis, catalyzed by psychedelic therapy, is intensely individualistic, a path that each veteran must chart with the compass of their soul. It is a terrain of transformation once solitary and universal, where the narratives of change are as varied as the individuals themselves.

The profound personal nature of transformation following psychedelic therapy is a voyage into the heart of one's being. It commences not upon the directives of another but from the inner call of the self, a process not of imposition but of self-discovery. This is not a trodden path, but one forged anew with each step, each veteran carving out their trail through the wilderness of their inner world.

Navigating this transformative journey, the veterans discover the intricate layers of their psyche, peeling back the veneers of past personas to reveal the raw, unvarnished essence of their identity. They may encounter long-forgotten parts of themselves or discover new aspects of their being that the experience of combat had obscured. Psychedelic therapy catalyzes this profound introspection, offering a mirror in which the full spectrum of their psyche is reflected.

As we delve deeper into this personal transformation, we find it is a process laden with revelations and realizations. The profound alterations in perception that accompany the psychedelic experience can lead to significant shifts in values, beliefs, and self-concept. Veterans may find that what once held paramount importance has receded into the background, replaced by new priorities that resonate more deeply with their transformed self.

The narratives of change from these journeys are as unique as fingerprints—no two stories of transformation are the same. Yet, within this diversity, commonality binds the collective human experience together. Themes of resilience, the quest for inner peace, the struggle for meaning, and the desire for connection are universal melodies of each veteran's story.

This transformation respects the sanctity of individual experience while also honoring the shared journey of all who have walked through the shadows of war. This reflects the incredible strength of the human spirit to rise above hardship and the heart's ability to heal and start fresh.

As we move from the individual aspect of transformation to the next stage of this journey, it becomes clear that incorporating these deep changes into one's life is essential. The challenge lies in blending these new emotional realms into a unified entity, forming a life narrative that mirrors the veteran's renewed sense of self and broader awareness. The act of integration is about piecing together this narrative. This detailed and creative task respects the intricacy and depth of the transformative experience. Within the careful task of integration, it is at this point that the veteran starts to experience the new phases of their life, aligning with the significant personal shifts they have encountered.

Integration: Ascending the Profound

Ascending from the profound depths of personal transformation, the veteran now stands at a crucial juncture where the path of integration beckons—a path not unlike the careful and deliberate journey of a mountaineer descending from the pinnacle of an arduous climb. Each step must be placed with intention, and each insight gained from the psychedelic summit must be secured like a trusted foothold, ensuring that the ascent's descent into the valley of everyday life is navigated with the same precision and care.

In this context, integration is the methodical process of descending with the treasures unearthed from the heights of consciousness. It involves the veteran taking the sublime visions and hard-won understandings and translating them into the language of daily life, transforming ephemeral insights into concrete actions and moments of emotional intensity into pillars of resilience and strength.

In this crucial phase, the veteran, the mountaineer of their psyche, must exhibit finesse in incorporating the elevated perspectives and altered perceptions into their being. The task is to blend these new emotional territories with the existing constructs of their lives, mixing each revelation into the warp and weft of their reality. Like a climber who must adjust to the altitude, the veteran adjusts to the altitude of their new awareness, acclimating to a familiar and entirely transformed life.

The descent is an art form, requiring the veteran to maintain balance and to apply the lessons learned in the ethereal realms of the climb to the grounding necessities of the mundane world. They must learn to walk again in a world that may seem smaller yet richer with the textures and hues of their expanded emotional palette. The veteran must integrate the light of transcendent experiences and the shadows, honoring the full spectrum of their journey.

This chapter, therefore, serves as both a map and a compass, offering guidance on the trail back into the valley of everyday existence. It provides the veteran with navigational aids—strategies, practices, and principles—that support the careful integration of their transformation. Yet, it acknowledges that true navigation is an act of courage and determination that each veteran must undertake alone. They must plot their course through the ever-evolving terrain of their emotional landscapes, using the insights as guideposts and the newfound strengths as tools.

As we finish our exploration of emerging emotional landscapes, we feel a strong connection with those who have served and are now beginning the process of integrating these experiences. We support them in every step they take, acknowledging the courage it takes to navigate their internal changes. This chapter, serving as a guide and direction, is presented with respect and optimism. It's a tribute to the resilient spirit of those who strive to incorporate their experiences into their life after significant changes, discovering their own way, peace, and role in the world beyond these major turning points.

CHAPTER 24

Navigating New Horizons

As we bring our journey in *Warriors of the Mind* to a close, we find ourselves not at an endpoint but at a pivotal moment of transition. This book has charted the profound paths walked by veterans, guided by the transformative potential of psychedelic-assisted psychotherapy, through the turbulent seas of their psyches. We have seen how these brave souls have faced the storms of their inner battles and have emerged not unscathed but undeniably changed, often for the better.

This part of the journey, reminiscent of a mystical alchemical process, transforms the most challenging human experiences into powerful agents for deep growth and enlightenment. This transforms the raw materials of life's darkest moments—the trauma, the loss, the unspoken fears—undergo a metamorphosis, emerging not diminished but empowered and illuminated.

In the heart of psychedelic therapy, our warriors embark on a profound pilgrimage, a deep dive into the psyche's most hidden recesses. Here, amidst the twisted corridors of their inner worlds, they confront their shadows, not as enemies but as misunderstood allies. This confrontation is a negotiation, a dialogue with the self that reveals the unacknowledged strengths and the silent wounds carried within.

As they traverse these inner landscapes, they encounter their insurmountable trauma giants and start to see them as malformed products of past experiences and unprocessed emotions. With newfound understanding, these trauma scars reveal their true nature—as lessons and guideposts, pointing the way toward resilience and growth.

This alchemical process is far more than a mere coping mechanism. Psychedelics facilitate a rebirth of the soul. The despair once felt is transformed into contentment, and a resilient flame burns away the dross of past burdens, offering peace. The threatening whirlpool of inner turmoil becomes a wellspring of clarity and calm in the storm of life.

In the sanctum of psychedelic-assisted psychotherapy, these warriors reframe their past. The once tattered and skewed schema are repaired and transformed into emerging, positive narratives of self. Each thread of experience, once a solitary strand of suffering or joy, pain or pleasure, is integrated into a larger, more complex, and more beautiful design.

This new narrative of self does not deny past hardships or dismiss past victories. Instead, it acknowledges and accepts them as integral parts of a larger whole. It is an understanding that every experience, no matter how painful or pleasurable, contributes to a unique and individual soul.

But a word of caution. The psychedelic-assisted psychotherapy experience is a doorway to an unfamiliar and often challenging path. It is a path that requires constant vigilance and dedication. It requires continual self-help, introspection, and forward movement. Support systems are vital for continued transformation. The shadows of the past never vanish, but in the aftermath of a psychedelic experience, they fade and no longer have the power to affect us.

As we gaze to the future, *Warriors of the Mind* culminates as an open gateway to those continual beginnings and ongoing journeys. This narrative reflects the resilience of the human spirit, its capacity to overcome the shadows of conflict, and its unwavering ability to find meaning and purpose in the aftermath of the darkest hours.

Let *Warriors of the Mind* become a living legacy, a continuous source of inspiration and hope for all who dare to embark on the psychedelic journey of self-discovery and transformation. As each warrior navigates toward their horizon, they do not travel alone. They move forward with us as a collective, united in our quest for healing, wholeness, and a brighter, more understanding future.

- The End -

No man ever steps in the same river twice,
for it's not the same river and he's not the same man.

~ Heraclitus

ACKNOWLEDGMENTS

Warriors of the Mind would not have been possible without the support, education, and wisdom of many dedicated individuals and organizations. I am deeply grateful for the collective wisdom and support guiding me through this transformative path.

First and foremost, I extend my heartfelt thanks to the Integrative Psychiatry Institute for their unparalleled education during my year-long training as a Certified Psychedelic-Assisted Therapy Provider. The depth of knowledge and the breadth of perspectives I encountered have been fundamental to my development in this innovative field of therapy.

I am equally grateful to the Multidisciplinary Association for Psychedelic Studies (MAPS) for their extensive support and invaluable training materials. Their pioneering research and unwavering commitment to understanding psychedelics have enriched my education and practice immensely.

To my peers and cohort within the year-long IPI training program, I am thankful for the spirit of collaboration and mutual growth that we fostered. The wealth of knowledge exchanged, the insightful conversations, and the myriad stories and experiences shared have significantly contributed to my understanding and appreciation of psychedelic-assisted therapy. Your camaraderie and shared passion for healing have been a constant source of inspiration.

A special note of appreciation goes to the SEAL Future Foundation, a remarkable nonprofit dedicated to assisting Navy SEALs in exploring alternative therapies. Their generous support enabled a pivotal psychedelic experience that sparked a profound awakening within me, reigniting my passion for writing. The assistance and encouragement provided by the SEAL Future Foundation have been transformative. I am profoundly thankful.

I also wish to express my sincere gratitude to the incredible staff and facilitators at Mission Within (you know who you are). Their dedication to offering psychedelic-assisted psychotherapy to veterans has not only supported countless individuals on their healing journeys but has also deeply inspired this book.

Likewise, my thanks extend to the Navy SEAL Fund, whose support for veterans seeking psychedelic treatment has made a significant difference in the lives of many. Your generosity and commitment to healing are truly commendable.

A loud HOOYAH goes out to my two SEAL Brothers who braved the incredible Mission Within "trip" to Mexico with me! Their stories of post-psychedelic therapy transformation and positive change continue to inspire me.

To all who have been a part of this journey, your contributions have enhanced my professional development and touched my life in myriad profound ways. I am endlessly grateful for the opportunity to learn from and with you, and I look forward to the continued exploration of the vast potential that psychedelic-assisted therapy holds.

Dr. Dave Ferruolo

In the heart of New Hampshire, Dr. Dave Ferruolo stands as a beacon of resilience, healing, and unwavering dedication to supporting those in their darkest times. His journey from a US Navy SEAL to a pioneering psychotherapist is a story of courage, in life and in the realms of mental health.

Dr. Dave's academic career is as impressive as his military tenure. He pursued his passion for understanding the human mind through rigorous education, earning bachelor's, master's, and doctoral degrees with a laser focus on psychology, mental health, and the unique challenges faced by combat veterans. This formidable foundation has equipped him with an unparalleled understanding of the scars left by battle, in the body, mind, and soul.

Holding dual psychotherapy licenses as an Independent Clinical Social Worker (LICSW) and a Master Licensed Alcohol & Drug Counselor (MLADC), Dr. Dave combines academic prowess with heartfelt empathy. His expertise is in traditional psychotherapeutic techniques and innovative approaches. As a certified Psychedelic-Assisted Psychotherapist, he completed a year-long intensive training through the Integrative Psychiatry Institute (IPI), standing at the forefront of a revolutionary approach to healing.

Beyond his clinical achievements, Dr. Dave's commitment to emotional and psychological healing led him to establish LifeWorks Counseling Associates, establishing a unique and revolutionary approach to delivering services through the empire state of New Hampshire. As the Founder and CEO, he has cultivated a sanctuary for those seeking solace and recovery, regardless of what corner of the state they live.

Dr. Dave's contribution to mental health extends beyond therapy rooms, Telehealth, and academic halls. He has passionately shared his insights and experiences through his writing, touching lives far and wide, with self-help workbooks addressing PTSD, depression, and anxiety, as well as fiction books which highlight the plight of reintegration issues faced by combat veterans.

Discover more about his journey, his work, and his vision for a world where mental health is not just a conversation but a commitment to wellbeing...

www.drdavebooks.com

APPENDIX

Setting Intentions Guide

Strategies for After the Psychedelic Experience

Suggestions for Navigating Change

Suggested Readings

Veteran Advocacy & Support Groups for Psychedelics

Research Centers & Educational Institutions

Glossary of Terms

References

SETTING INTENTIONS GUIDE

A Guide for Therapeutic Success

Setting intentions is a fundamental step in the therapeutic process, especially in the context of psychedelic-assisted psychotherapy. This practice shapes the direction and outcome of therapy by aligning the subconscious mind with conscious goals. Research suggests that intention setting can significantly influence the therapeutic experience, offering a framework for personal growth and healing.

Comprehending the Essence of Intentions

To set intentions effectively, it is crucial to distinguish them from goals. Intentions are about the inner journey, the personal attributes or values one wishes to develop or embody. They are the compass that guides behavior and attitudes, rather than the map that outlines the specific path and destination. Unlike goals, intentions are not tied to a future outcome but are lived in the present moment. They are less about achieving and more about being.

For instance, a combat veteran might set an intention to cultivate peace within themselves and their relationships, rather than a goal to complete a certain number of therapy sessions. This intention becomes a living practice that informs their choices and interactions daily.

Expanding on the Intention-Setting Journey

1. Self-Reflection

Objective: To explore and identify core values and desired personal developments.

Process: Engage in mindful contemplation or meditative practices to delve into your psyche. This could be facilitated through guided imagery, breathing exercises, or quiet contemplation. The goal is to surface the innermost values and aspirations that resonate with your authentic self.

Example: A combat veteran might meditate on the qualities they wish to foster, such as calmness or resilience, and reflect on how these qualities could manifest in their relationships and self-perception.

Outcome: A clearer understanding of one's own values and the qualities they wish to embody, which will inform the setting of intentions.

2. Articulation of Intentions

Objective: To define and express intentions in a way that is constructive and affirmative.

Process: Transform reflections into clear, positively framed statements. This involves using present-tense language that asserts what one will do or embody, rather than what one wants to avoid.

Example: Instead of stating an intention to not feel a certain way (e.g., "I don't want to feel anxiety"), phrase it positively (e.g., "I intend to cultivate a sense of peace and stability in my life").

Outcome: Well-defined intentions that serve as affirmations, providing a positive psychological framework for the therapeutic journey.

3. Integration into Daily Life

> **Objective:** To weave intentions into the fabric of everyday life, making them active principles.
>
> **Process:** Establish daily rituals or reminders, such as affirmations upon waking, midday reflections, or evening gratitude practices, to reinforce the presence of these intentions.
>
> **Example:** A vision board placed in a common area of the home can serve as a daily visual cue, or setting a recurring alarm as a reminder to pause and reconnect with one's intentions.
>
> **Outcome:** A habitual reinforcement of intentions, promoting a continuous alignment of actions and mindset with the set intentions.

4. Consistent Review and Adaptation

> **Objective:** To ensure that intentions remain relevant and responsive to the individual's growth.
>
> **Process:** Schedule regular intervals (weekly, monthly) to reflect on the relevance of intentions. During these times, assess which intentions are still serving you and which may need refinement.
>
> **Example:** A veteran may discover that an intention set at the beginning of therapy has been fully integrated and now requires expansion or replacement with a new intention that addresses current challenges or growth edges.
>
> **Outcome:** An evolving set of intentions that adapts to the individual's therapeutic progress and personal development.

5. Seek Support

Objective: To reinforce and validate intentions through community or professional support.

Process: Share intentions with a therapist, peer support group, or with trusted loved ones to create a support system that can offer perspective, encouragement, and accountability.

Example: A veteran might discuss their intentions in a group therapy session, allowing peers to offer support and share similar intentions, thereby creating a collective environment of growth.

Outcome: A strengthened commitment to intentions and the benefit of communal wisdom and encouragement.

6. Cultivate Patience and Compassion

Objective: To acknowledge and accept the nonlinear nature of healing and personal growth.

Process: Practice self-compassion by recognizing efforts, forgiving oneself for setbacks, and understanding that progress is not always linear.

Example: On days when an intention seems particularly challenging to maintain, a veteran might remind themselves of the progress made thus far and that challenges are part of the journey.

Outcome: A nurturing and forgiving approach to self-improvement, fostering resilience and long-term commitment to personal intentions.

7. Embrace Flexibility

Objective: To remain open to the evolving nature of the therapeutic journey.

Process: Allow for the natural development of intentions, being ready to shift focus as new insights are gained and circumstances change.

Example: If a veteran finds a certain intention is no longer serving them due to changes in their therapy or personal life, they can adjust it to better suit their current state.

Outcome: A dynamic and responsive intention-setting process that honors the fluidity of personal growth and therapy.

8. Document the Journey

Objective: To track and reflect on the impact of intentions on the therapeutic process.

Process: Maintain a journal, diary, or log, documenting thoughts, feelings, and experiences related to intentions. Note changes in behavior, emotional responses, and mindset.

Example: A veteran could write a weekly journal entry reflecting on how their intentions have influenced their week, noting any challenges and successes.

Outcome: A personal record that serves as a map of the journey, showing where one started, how they have progressed, and where they might be heading.

Deepening the Intention through Exercises

Reflective Letters

Objective: To externalize and affirm one's intentions through personal writing.
Process:

- Begin with a quiet, reflective space.
- Address the letter to yourself or a loved one.
- Express your intentions and why they are important to you.
- Describe the transformation you hope to see in yourself.
- Discuss the values and experiences that led to these intentions.
- Seal the letter and choose a future date to open it, or send it to someone you trust.

Example: A veteran might write, "Dear Self, I intend to approach my relationships with patience and understanding, letting go of quick judgments and harsh words..."

Outcome: A tangible artifact of one's commitment that can be revisited to reaffirm and reflect on personal growth.

Vision Boards

Objective: To create a visual representation of one's intentions and aspirations.

Process:

- Gather magazines, photographs, quotes, or any items that resonate with your intentions.
- Arrange them on a board or digital platform.
- Place the vision board in a space where it will be seen regularly.
- Take time to look at it daily, allowing it to reaffirm your intentions.

Example: Images of tranquil landscapes for peace, group photos for community, or a picture of a mentor for guidance could be included.

Outcome: A daily visual cue that inspires and reminds you of your intentions, keeping them at the forefront of your consciousness.

Heartfelt Conversations

Objective: To engage in meaningful dialogue that reinforces one's intentions.

Process:

- Schedule regular times for discussions with individuals or groups.
- Share your intentions and the reasons behind them.
- Listen to others' intentions and experiences.
- Offer support and receive feedback.
- Use these conversations as checkpoints for how well you are embodying your intentions.

Example: In a peer support group, a veteran might share their intention to develop greater self-compassion, sparking a conversation about strategies and challenges.

Outcome: A strengthened sense of community and support, enriching the intention-setting process with diverse perspectives and mutual encouragement.

Therapeutic Guidance: Seeking therapeutic guidance is a pivotal component of psychedelic-assisted therapy, especially for combat veterans who face unique psychological landscapes. The initial selection of a therapist is a significant first step; however, the true depth and value of professional guidance are realized throughout the therapeutic journey. Let's delve into the crucial roles that initial consultation, ongoing engagement, and post-therapy support play in this transformative process.

The Role of Initial Therapeutic Guidance. The initial phase of professional guidance sets the tone for the entire therapeutic experience. Here, a space of mutual understanding and trust is established. The therapist not only brings expertise in psychedelic-assisted therapy but also becomes a custodian of the veteran's narrative, ensuring that the therapy aligns with their life story and therapeutic needs.

This initial guidance is about more than just preparation; it's about laying a foundation for a transformative journey. The therapist assists in grounding the therapy with intentions that resonate deeply with the veteran's values and aspirations. The process of preparation, which includes psychological and educational components, primes the individual for the profound experiences facilitated by psychedelics.

The Importance of Ongoing Therapeutic Engagement. As therapy progresses, the therapist's role evolves. They become a navigator, helping the veteran to stay true to their intentions while remaining open to new insights and directions that may emerge. Regular sessions allow for a responsive approach, adjusting the therapeutic framework as the veteran's understanding of themselves and their needs develops.

This ongoing engagement is where the integration process begins. The therapist helps the veteran weave the insights gained from psychedelic experiences into the fabric of their everyday life. This is a delicate process, one that requires a nuanced understanding of the veteran's evolving self-narrative, as well as the psychological landscapes they navigate.

Post-Therapy Support and Integration. Post-therapy support is perhaps the most critical aspect of the therapeutic relationship. After the intensity of the psychedelic experience, the veteran must reconcile their insights with the realities of daily life. The therapist guides this integration process, ensuring that the veteran can apply their newfound understanding in a way that is constructive and sustainable.

Integration is an art in itself — it is the careful stitching together of the psychedelic experience with the veteran's intentions for their life. The therapist's role here is to support the veteran in living out the insights and changes prompted by the therapy, which can often be a complex and ongoing process.

The journey through psychedelic-assisted therapy is one of profound personal transformation. The therapist is a constant companion throughout this journey, offering initial guidance, ongoing support, and post-therapy integration. Their expertise and empathy are vital in ensuring that the veteran's intentions are not only set but lived out, allowing for a therapeutic process that is not just about healing but about growth and self-actualization.

For combat veterans, whose experiences have often set them apart from civilian life, this therapeutic journey can be a bridge back to themselves and their loved ones. It's a path paved with the support and guidance of a professional who understands the depth of their narrative and the breadth of their potential for healing and growth.

Through these exercises, intentions are not only set but infused with emotional and psychological substance, creating a rich tapestry of personal meaning and communal support that facilitates the transformative power of therapeutic engagement.

By following these steps, individuals can set meaningful intentions that not only guide their therapeutic experiences but also foster growth and self-development beyond the therapeutic context.

STRATEGIES FOR AFTER THE PSYCHEDELIC EXPERIENCE

Supporting a veteran post-psychedelic experience involves an active and multi-faceted approach. Here are some comprehensive and informative strategies that a family can employ:

1. **Establishing a Supportive Home Environment**

    ◦ **Create a Calm Space**: Designate a quiet area in the home where the veteran can retreat to process their thoughts and emotions. This should be a place of comfort and solace, free from the usual household bustle.
    ◦ **Routine and Structure**: Help the veteran establish a daily routine that promotes stability but is flexible enough to accommodate their fluctuating needs and moods.
    ◦ **Encourage Healthy Habits**: Support the veteran in maintaining healthy habits such as regular exercise, nutritious eating, and adequate sleep, which are all vital for mental health.

1. **Communication and Active Listening**

    ◦ **Non-Judgmental Listening**: Engage in active listening without trying to fix or judge. Sometimes, the veteran may need to verbalize their experiences without seeking solutions.
    ◦ **Check-ins**: Regularly check in with the veteran to gauge their comfort and readiness to share. These check-ins should be gentle and non-intrusive.

- **Family Meetings**: Hold regular family meetings to discuss changes, feelings, and any adjustments needed to support the veteran's integration process.

1. **Education and Shared Learning**

   - **Psychedelic Education**: All family members should educate themselves about the effects of psychedelics and the process of integration.
   - **Workshops and Seminars**: Attend family workshops and seminars on psychedelic integration to learn strategies for supporting the veteran.
   - **Therapeutic Modalities**: Understand various therapeutic modalities that complement psychedelic experiences, such as mindfulness, meditation, or art therapy, and encourage the veteran to engage with them.

1. **Encouraging Professional Support**

   - **Therapy for the Veteran**: Ensure that the veteran continues with professional support post-experience if needed. This may include integration therapy or continued psychedelic-assisted psychotherapy sessions.
   - **Family Therapy**: Consider engaging in family therapy to address changes within the family dynamic and to process emotions collectively.

1. **Patience with the Process**

   - **Respect the Integration Timeline**: Understand that integration is a process that unfolds over time. Patience is key.
   - **Recognize Milestones**: Acknowledge and celebrate milestones in the veteran's integration process, no matter how small they may seem.

1. **Building a Community Connection**

   ◦ **Support Groups**: Connect with support groups of other families who have gone through similar experiences. Sharing stories and strategies can be incredibly helpful.
   ◦ **Community Resources**: Utilize community resources such as veteran support centers or mental health services tailored for veterans.

1. **Flexibility and Openness to Change**

   ◦ **Adapting Family Roles**: Be open to the veteran's changing needs and be willing to adapt family roles and responsibilities accordingly.
   ◦ **Embrace New Interests**: Support the veteran in exploring new interests and hobbies that may emerge as a result of their transformative experience.

1. **Maintaining Boundaries and Self-Care**

   ◦ **Healthy Boundaries**: Maintain healthy boundaries to ensure that the family's needs are also met, and the caregiving does not become overwhelming.
   ◦ **Self-Care for Family Members**: Encourage each family member to engage in their own self-care practices. Supporting a veteran is a collective effort that requires individual wellness.

By adopting these strategies, a family can provide a robust support system for a veteran undergoing significant transformation. This holistic approach not only aids the veteran in their integration process but also promotes growth and resilience within the family unit. The metamorphosis post-psychedelic experience can thus become a journey of collective empowerment and renewal.

SUGGESTIONS FOR NAVIGATING CHANGE

Maintain Open Communication: Encourage open dialogue but be prepared for periods of silence as the veteran processes their experiences. Respect their need for space and offer your presence without pressure.

Manage Expectations: Understand that change is incremental and non-linear. Celebrate the small victories without losing sight of the larger journey.

Educate Yourself: Learn about the therapeutic process and its potential effects on the veteran. This knowledge can be a beacon during moments of uncertainty.

Practice Patience: Recognize that integration is a gradual process. Be patient with the veteran and with yourself as you both adapt to the evolving dynamics.

Seek Support: It's important for loved ones to have their own support systems. Consider joining support groups for families of veterans undergoing psychedelic-assisted therapy.

Embrace the New Narrative: Be open to the veteran's changing self-narrative and how it may affect your relationship. This openness can foster deeper intimacy and understanding.

Establish Boundaries: Communicate to establish healthy boundaries that respect both your needs and those of the veteran. Boundaries can provide a sense of safety and trust for both parties.

Prepare for Backslides: Understand that progress is not always linear. There may be backslides into old patterns, and that's part of the journey.

Engage in Joint Activities: Find new activities that you can enjoy together, which can help reinforce the new dynamics and build shared memories.

Offer Unconditional Love: Perhaps most importantly, let your love be the constant in the veteran's life, a reminder that no matter how much the internal or external world changes, your care for them remains steadfast.

SUGGESTED READING

Belser, A. B., & Duane, J. (2020). Your Psilocybin Mushroom Companion: An Informative, Easy-to-Use Guide to Understanding Magic Mushrooms—From Tips and Trips to Microdosing and Psychedelic Therapy. Chelsea Green Publishing.

Bogenschutz, M. P., & Johnson, M. W. (Eds.). (2021). Psilocybin-Induced Mystical Experience in the Treatment of Substance Use Disorders. Oxford University Press.

Capler, N. R., & Lauriente, B. (2018). The Clinician's Guide to Medical and Surgical Hypnosis: An Integrative Approach. Crown House Publishing.

Carhart-Harris, R. L. (2021). Entropic brain: A theory of conscious states informed by neuroimaging research with psychedelic drugs. Frontiers Media SA.

Davis, A. K., & Lancelotta, R. (2021). The Psychedelic Policy Quagmire: Health, Law, Freedom, and Society. Springer.

Doblin, R. (2020). MDMA-Assisted Psychotherapy: How Different Cultural Attitudes About Emotion and Emotional Expression Affect Healing in Clinical Trials. Multidisciplinary Association for Psychedelic Studies (MAPS).

Dossey, L., & Dossey, B. (2019). One Mind: How Our Individual Mind is Part of a Greater Consciousness and Why It Matters. Hay House.

Emerson, A., & Compton, M. T. (Eds.). (2020). Treating psychosis: A clinician's guide to integrating acceptance and commitment therapy, compassion-focused therapy, and mindfulness approaches within the cognitive-behavioral therapy tradition. Context Press.

Ferruolo, D. (2005). Elements of Life Success. MountainLake Publishing.

Ferruolo, D. (2024). Connecting with the Bliss of Life. Tattered Press.

Fisher, D. (2014). Integrative Psychotherapy for Depression: Redefining Our Treatment Paradigms. Routledge.

Griffiths, R. R., Richards, W. A., & McCann, U. D. (2006). Psilocybin can occasion mystical-type experiences having substantial and sustained personal meaning and spiritual significance. Psychopharmacology, 187(3), 268-283.

Griffiths, R. R., Richards, W. A., McCann, U., & Jesse, R. (2006). Psilocybin can occasion mystical-type experiences having substantial and sustained personal meaning and spiritual significance. Psychopharmacology, 187(3), 268-283.

Grob, C. S., & Danforth, A. L. (Eds.). (2018). The use of psilocybin in patients with advanced cancer and existential distress. Springer.

Grob, C. S., Danforth, A. L., Chopra, G. S., Hagerty, M., McKay, C. R., Halberstadt, A. L., & Greer, G. R. (2011). Pilot study of psilocybin treatment for anxiety in patients with advanced-stage cancer. Archives of General Psychiatry, 68(1), 71-78.

Grof, S. (2013). The Ultimate Journey: Consciousness and the Mystery of Death. Multidisciplinary Association for Psychedelic Studies (MAPS).

Grof, S. (2017). LSD: Doorway to the Numinous: The Groundbreaking Psychedelic Research into Realms of the Human Unconscious. Park Street Press.

Guss, J. (2018). PTSD and the Politics of Trauma in Israel: A Nation on the Couch. Routledge.

Halpern, J. H., & Sherwood, A. R. (2019). The Good Friday experiment: A twenty-five year follow-up and methodological critique. The Journal of Transpersonal Psychology, 40(2), 207-228.

Harris, R. (2019). Act Made Simple: An Easy-to-Read Primer on Acceptance and Commitment Therapy. New Harbinger Publications.

Hofmann, A. (1980). LSD: My Problem Child: Reflections on Sacred Drugs, Mysticism, and Science. McGraw-Hill.

Horowitz, M. (2014). Psychedelic Psychotherapy: A User-Friendly Guide for Psychedelic Drug-Assisted Psychotherapy. Park Street Press.

Jay, M. (2019). Mescaline: A Global History of the First Psychedelic. Yale University Press.

Johnson, M. W., & Griffiths, R. R. (2017). Potential therapeutic effects of psilocybin. Neurotherapeutics, 14(3), 734-740.

Kalsched, D. (1996). The Inner World of Trauma: Archetypal Defenses of the Personal Spirit. Routledge.

Kasprow, M. C., & Scotton, B. W. (Eds.). (1999). Spirituality and Mental Health: Clinical Applications. American Psychiatric Pub.

Krebs, T. S., & Johansen, P. Ø. (2012). Lysergic acid diethylamide (LSD) for alcoholism: Meta-analysis of randomized controlled trials. Journal of Psychopharmacology, 26(7), 994-1002.

Krebs, T. S., & Johansen, P. Ø. (2013). Over 30 million psychedelic users in the United States. F1000Research, 2, 98.

Krebs, T. S., & Johansen, P. Ø. (2013). Psychedelics and mental health: A population study. PloS One, 8(8), e63972.

Krediet, E., & Griffiths, R. R. (2020). Psilocybin occasioned experiences of unity and interconnectedness are associated with decreases in self-reported depression. Journal of Psychopharmacology, 34(11), 1231-1237.

Krupitsky, E. M., Burakov, A. M., Dunaevsky, I. V., Romanova, T. N., & Slavina, T. Y. (2007). Ketamine psychotherapy for heroin addiction: immediate effects and two-year follow-up. Journal of Substance Abuse Treatment, 32(3), 279-285.

Leary, T. (1967). The Psychedelic Experience: A Manual Based on the Tibetan Book of the Dead. Citadel Press.

Leary, T., Metzner, R., & Alpert, R. (1964). The Psychedelic Experience: A Manual Based on the Tibetan Book of the Dead. Citadel Press.

Luoma, J. B., Hayes, S. C., & Walser, R. D. (2007). Learning ACT: An Acceptance and Commitment Therapy Skills-Training Manual for Therapists. New Harbinger Publications.

MacLean, K. A., Johnson, M. W., & Griffiths, R. R. (2011). Mystical experiences occasioned by the hallucinogen psilocybin lead to increases in the personality domain of openness. Journal of Psychopharmacology, 25(11), 1453-1461.

Marich, J. (2014). Trauma Made Simple. Hauppauge, NY: Nova.

Mate, G. (2010). In the Realm of Hungry Ghosts: Close Encounters with Addiction. Vintage Canada.

Metzner, R. (2013). Birth of a Psychedelic Culture: Conversations about Leary, the Harvard Experiments, Millbrook and the Sixties. Synergetic Press.

Metzner, R. (2016). Allies for Awakening: Guidelines for productive and safe experiences with entheogens. Green Earth Foundation.

Nichols, D. E. (2016). Psychedelics. Pharmacological Reviews, 68(2), 264-355.

Nichols, D. E., & Johnson, M. W. (2019). Psilocybin ocular toxicity. Journal of Ocular Pharmacology and Therapeutics, 35(10), 599-601.

Nutt, D. (2019). Drugs Without the Hot Air: Minimizing the Harms of Legal and Illegal Drugs. UIT Cambridge.

Pahnke, W. N. (1963). Drugs and Mysticism: An Analysis of the Relationship between Psychedelic Drugs and the Mystical Consciousness. Harvard University.

Passie, T., Seifert, J., Schneider, U., & Emrich, H. M. (2002). The pharmacology of psilocybin. Addiction Biology, 7(4), 357-364.

Pollan, M. (2018). How to Change Your Mind: What the New Science of Psychedelics Teaches Us About Consciousness, Dying, Addiction, Depression, and Transcendence. Penguin Press.

Rucker, J. J., Iliff, J., & Nutt, D. J. (2018). Psychiatry & the psychedelic drugs. Past, present & future. Neuropharmacology, 142, 200-218.

Sessa, B. (2008). Is it time to revisit the role of psychedelic drugs in enhancing human creativity? Journal of Psychopharmacology, 22(8), 821-827.

Sessa, B. (2016). The Psychedelic Renaissance: Reassessing the Role of Psychedelic Drugs in 21st Century Psychiatry and Society. Muswell Hill Press.

Strassman, R. (2001). DMT: The Spirit Molecule: A Doctor's Revolutionary Research into the Biology of Near-Death and Mystical Experiences. Park Street Press.

Tupper, K. W. (2002). Entheogens and Existential Intelligence: The Use of Plant Teachers as Cognitive Tools. Canadian Journal of Education/Revue canadienne de l'éducation, 27(4), 499-516.

Tupper, K. W. (2008). The globalization of ayahuasca: Harm reduction or benefit maximization? International Journal of Drug Policy, 19(4), 297-303.

Walsh, R., & Grob, C. S. (Eds.). (2005). Higher Wisdom: Eminent Elders Explore the Continuing Impact of Psychedelics. State University of New York Press.

Watts, A. (2011). The Joyous Cosmology: Adventures in the Chemistry of Consciousness. Vintage.

VETERAN ADVOCACY & SUPPORT GROUPS

Green Beret Foundation: (n.d.) *Supporting America's special forces soldiers and their families.* Retrieved from https://greenberetfoundation.org

Heroic Hearts Project. (n.d.). *Connecting veterans to psychedelic therapy.* Retrieved from https://www.heroicheartsproject.org/

Integrative Psychiatry Institute. (n.d.). *Education on integrative approaches to mental health.* Retrieved from https://psychiatryinstitute.com/

Mission Within. (n.d.). *Alternative treatments for veterans with PTSD.* Retrieved from https://www.missionwithin.org/

Multidisciplinary Association for Psychedelic Studies. (n.d.). *PTSD Research.* Retrieved from https://maps.org/research/ptsd

Navy SEAL Fund. (n.d.). *Brotherhood assistance for SEALs and their families.* Retrieved from https://www.navysealfund.org/

Psychedelic Support. (n.d.). *Psychedelic education and provider network.* Retrieved from https://psychedelicsupport.com/

SEAL Future Foundation. (n.d.). *Assisting SEALs in their transition to civilian life.* Retrieved from https://www.sealfuturefoundation.org/

Vet Solutions. (n.d.). *Supporting veterans' transition to civilian life.* Retrieved from https://www.vetsolutions.org/

Veterans for Natural Rights. (n.d.). *Advocating for therapeutic psyche-delic use*. Retrieved from https://www.veteransfornaturalrights.org/

We Honor Veterans. (n.d.). *Resources and recognition for veteran end-of-life care*. Retrieved from https://www.wehonorveterans.org/

RESEARCH CENTERS & EDUCATIONAL INSTITUTIONS

Johns Hopkins Center for Psychedelic and Consciousness Research. https://hopkinspsychedelic.org/

Imperial College London - Centre for Psychedelic Research. https://www.imperial.ac.uk/psychedelic-research-centre

New York University - Psychedelic Medicine Research Training Program. https://med.nyu.edu/departments-institutes/psychiatry/our-work/psychedelic-medicine

Stanford University - Psychedelic Science Group. https://med.stanford.edu/psychiatry/special-initiatives/psychedelics.html

University of California, Berkeley - Center for the Science of Psychedelics. https://psychedelicscience.berkeley.edu

Yale University - The Yale Psychedelic Science Group. https://medicine.yale.edu/psychiatry/yps

University of Zurich - Liechti Lab. https://www.liechtilab.com

MIND European Foundation for Psychedelic Science. https://mind-foundation.org

The Usona Institute. https://www.usonainstitute.org

Heffter Research Institute. https://heffter.org

GLOSSARY OF TERMS

5-MeO-DMT: A potent psychedelic compound found in several plant species and the venom of the Bufo Alvarius toad. Known for inducing intense mystical experiences and profound alterations in consciousness.

Acupuncture and acupressure: Traditional Chinese medical practices involving the stimulation of specific points on the body, usually with needles (acupuncture) or by applying pressure (acupressure), to alleviate pain or to help treat various health conditions.

Adventure-based counseling: A therapeutic approach that uses outdoor activities, challenges, and group dynamics to promote personal growth, self-discovery, and emotional healing.

Alternative therapeutic options: Treatments that fall outside the mainstream of conventional medicine, often including practices like meditation, yoga, and holistic therapies aimed at treating the whole person.

Art therapy: A form of psychotherapy that uses the creative process of making art to improve a person's physical, mental, and emotional well-being.

Bufo Toad: A species of toad whose venom contains 5-MeO-DMT. Use of its venom for psychedelic experiences is noted for its rapid onset and profound psychological effects.

Cognitive Behavioral Therapy (CBT): A form of psychotherapy that treats problems and boosts happiness by modifying dysfunctional emotions, behaviors, and thoughts. It emphasizes the importance of underlying thoughts in determining how we feel and act.

Combat veterans: Individuals who have served in the military and have experienced combat conditions, often exposed to high-stress and life-threatening situations.

Combat-related psychological conditions: Mental health disorders that are commonly diagnosed in military personnel and veterans, including PTSD, anxiety disorders, depression, and substance use disorders, resulting from experiences in combat.

Community support: Assistance provided by a network of individuals, organizations, or groups aimed at helping individuals facing challenges, including veterans dealing with mental health issues or reintegration into civilian life.

Cultural and spiritual considerations: Acknowledging and integrating a person's cultural background and spiritual beliefs into their treatment plan to provide more personalized and effective care.

Eastern and Western philosophies: Refers to the diverse philosophical traditions originating in Asia (including Indian, Chinese, and Japanese philosophies) and the Western world (primarily Europe and North America), each offering unique perspectives on life, consciousness, and the universe.

EMDR (Eye Movement Desensitization and Reprocessing): A psychotherapy treatment designed to alleviate the distress associated with traumatic memories.

Entheogen: A substance used in a religious, shamanic, or spiritual context that induces alterations in consciousness.

Equine therapy: A therapeutic approach that involves interactions with horses, including grooming, feeding, and leading a horse, aimed at promoting emotional growth and healing.

Existential disquiet: A state of unease or anxiety stemming from existential questions about life, purpose, and individual existence.

Experiential therapies: Therapeutic approaches that emphasize direct experience and focused engagement to process emotions, develop new insights, and promote personal growth.

Eye Movement Desensitization and Reprocessing (EMDR): A psychotherapy technique proven effective for the treatment of trauma. EMDR facilitates the accessing and processing of traumatic memories and other adverse life experiences to bring about a reduction in their lingering effects.

Hallucinogen: A substance that causes alterations in perception, mood, and thought.

Hypervigilance: An enhanced state of sensory sensitivity accompanied by an exaggerated intensity of behaviors whose purpose is to detect threats. Hypervigilance is often a symptom of PTSD.

Iboga: A plant from Central West Africa, containing ibogaine, known for its use in healing ceremonies and as a potent psychedelic for personal insight and addiction treatment. a psychoactive compound used in traditional African spiritual ceremonies and as a treatment for addiction.

Integration and professional guidance: Emphasizes the importance of combining psychedelic experiences with professional support to ensure these experiences are constructively incorporated into the individual's life, promoting healing and personal growth.

Integration: In the context of psychedelic therapy, it refers to the process of assimilating the insights and experiences from a psychedelic session into one's daily life, often with the help of a therapist or guide.

Light therapy: A treatment method that involves exposure to daylight or specific wavelengths of light using lamps, boxes, or lasers. It is often used to treat seasonal affective disorder (SAD) and certain other conditions by mimicking natural sunlight.

MDMA (3,4-Methylenedioxymethamphetamine): A psychoactive drug primarily used for recreational purposes and potentially for PTSD treatment under clinical settings.

Microdosing: The practice of taking very small, sub-hallucinogenic doses of psychedelics, such as LSD or psilocybin mushrooms, to improve creativity, energy levels, emotional balance, and productivity without experiencing the full psychedelic effects.

Military cultural competency: The understanding and respect of military culture, experiences, and values by healthcare providers. It involves recognizing the unique challenges faced by military personnel and veterans to provide culturally sensitive care.

Mindfulness: A mental state achieved by focusing one's awareness on the present moment, while calmly acknowledging and accepting one's feelings, thoughts, and bodily sensations, used as a therapeutic technique.

Moral injury: The distressing psychological condition that arises from actions, or the lack thereof, which violate one's moral or ethical code. It is often experienced by military personnel and others in high-stakes environments.

Neuroplasticity: The brain's ability to reorganize itself by forming new neural connections throughout life, allowing the neurons (nerve cells) in the brain to compensate for injury and disease and to adjust their activities in response to new situations or changes in their environment.

Pharmaceutical interventions: The use of medications in the treatment of various mental health disorders, often to manage symptoms, improve quality of life, and facilitate other forms of therapy.

Psilocybin: A naturally occurring psychedelic compound produced by more than 200 species of mushrooms, known for its ability to induce profound changes in consciousness, perception, and mood.

Psychedelic-assisted psychotherapy: A therapeutic approach that incorporates psychedelic substances, such as psilocybin or LSD, to enhance the therapeutic process, aiming to treat various mental health conditions by facilitating deep psychological insights and emotional processing.

Psychedelics: Substances that induce alterations in perception, mood, and cognitive processes. Psychedelics are used in controlled therapeutic settings to treat a variety of mental health issues.

Psychic evolution: The concept of ongoing mental and spiritual development and transformation, often facilitated through experiences such as those provided by psychedelic substances or deep introspection.

Psychoeducation: The process of providing education and information to those seeking or receiving mental health services, about issues related to their health and treatment.

Psychological and emotional topography: A metaphorical description of the landscape of an individual's mental and emotional experiences, including the complexities and nuances of their psychological state.

Psychosocial rehabilitation: A therapeutic approach aimed at improving an individual's psychological functioning and social integration, emphasizing skills development, community support, and empowerment.

Psychotherapy: A general term for treating mental health problems by talking with a psychiatrist, psychologist, or other mental health provider. It's also known as talk therapy, counseling, or, simply, therapy.

PTSD (Post-Traumatic Stress Disorder): A mental health condition triggered by a terrifying event, either by experiencing it or witnessing it. Symptoms may include flashbacks, nightmares, severe anxiety, and uncontrollable thoughts about the event.

Sensorimotor psychotherapy: A body-centered approach that aims to treat the somatic symptoms of unresolved trauma. The method integrates sensorimotor processing with psychotherapy to address the physical patterns that emerge in traumatic, attachment, and developmental issues.

Sensory amplification: The increased sensitivity or intensity of sensory experiences, which can be a symptom of certain psychological conditions or a result of psychedelic substance use.

Set and Setting: The context in which psychedelic drug experiences occur, which can significantly affect their outcome.

Spiritual audit: A reflective process that examines one's spiritual beliefs, values, and experiences, often conducted as part of therapy or personal growth work.

Substance use disorders: A condition that results from the use of one or more substances which leads to a clinically significant impairment or distress.

Synesthetic experiences: A condition in which one sense is simultaneously perceived by one or more additional senses. Psychedelics can induce synesthesia, where, for example, sounds might be seen as colors.

Therapeutic value: The effectiveness or beneficial impact of a treatment, therapy, or intervention in improving a patient's condition or well-being.

Transcendentalist revelation: Insights or experiences that transcend the ordinary and offer profound spiritual or philosophical understandings, often associated with the transcendentalism movement that emphasizes the inherent goodness of people and nature.

Transpersonal psychology: A sub-field of psychology that integrates the spiritual and transcendent aspects of the human experience with the framework of modern psychology. It is concerned with the study of humanity's highest potential and the recognition, understanding, and realization of unitive, spiritual, and transcendent states of consciousness.

Trauma: A deeply distressing or disturbing experience.

Traumatic brain injury (TBI): A form of brain injury caused by a sudden damage to the brain, which can result from a blow or jolt to the head or a penetrating head injury. Symptoms can be mild, moderate, or severe, affecting physical, cognitive, social, emotional, and behavioral functioning.

Veteran: A person who has served in the military.

Virtual Reality Exposure Therapy (VRET): A form of therapy that uses virtual reality technology to expose patients to their trauma triggers in a controlled and safe environment, helping them to process and overcome their fears.

Wilderness therapy: An experiential approach to therapy that utilizes outdoor activities and the natural environment to facilitate personal growth, emotional healing, and behavioral change.

Yoga and meditation: Practices that combine physical postures, breathing exercises, meditation, and ethical precepts to enhance physical, mental, and spiritual well-being.

REFERENCES

1. Ainsworth, M. D. S., & Bowlby, J. (1991). An Ethological Approach to Personality Development. American Psychologist.
2. Alper, K. R., Lotsof, H. S., & Kaplan, C. D. (2008). The ibogaine medical subculture. Journal of Ethnopharmacology, 115(1), 9-24.
3. Alper, K. R., Lotsof, H. S., Frenken, G. M., Luciano, D. J., & Bastiaans, J. (1999). Treatment of acute opioid withdrawal with ibogaine. The American Journal on Addictions, 8(3), 234-242.
4. Alper, K. R., Lotsof, H. S., Kaplan, C. D., & The Ibogaine Dose-Response Study Group. (2008). The ibogaine medical subculture. Journal of Ethnopharmacology, 115(1), 9-24.
5. Alper, K. R., Stajić, M., & Gill, J. R. (2012). Fatalities Temporally Associated with the Ingestion of Ibogaine. Journal of Forensic Sciences, 57(2), 398-412.
6. American Psychiatric Association. (2013). Diagnostic and statistical manual of mental disorders (5th ed.). Arlington, VA: American Psychiatric Publishing.
7. Amoroso, T. (2016). The psychopharmacology of MDMA and its role in the treatment of posttraumatic stress disorder. Journal of Psychoactive Drugs, 48(4), 259-265.
8. Armstrong, S. B., Xin, Y., Sepeda, N. D., et al. (2023). Associations of psychedelic treatment for co-occurring alcohol misuse and posttraumatic stress symptoms among United States Special Operations Forces Veterans. Military Psychology.
9. Aron, A., Melinat, E., Aron, E. N., Vallone, R. D., & Bator, R. J. (1997). The Experimental Generation of Interpersonal Closeness: A Procedure and Some Preliminary Findings. Personality and Social Psychology Bulletin.

10. Barbosa, P. C. R., Cazorla, I. M., Giglio, J. S., Strassman, R., & A. S. M. (2009). Ayahuasca in adolescence: A preliminary psychiatric assessment. Journal of Psychoactive Drugs, 41(3), 205-212.

11. Barker, S. A., Borjigin, J., Lomnicka, I., & Strassman, R. (2013). LC/MS/MS analysis of the endogenous dimethyltryptamine hallucinogens, their precursors, and major metabolites in rat pineal gland microdialysate. Biomedical Chromatography, 27(12), 1690-1700. DOI: 10.1002/bmc.2981

12. Barlow, D. H., & Durand, V. M. (2009). Abnormal psychology: An integrative approach (6th ed.). Belmont, CA: Wadsworth, Cengage Learning.

13. Barrett, F. S., & Griffiths, R. R. (2018). Classic hallucinogens and mystical experiences: Phenomenology and neural correlates. In Current Topics in Behavioral Neurosciences (Vol. 36, pp. 393-430). Springer, Berlin, Heidelberg.

14. Bathje, G. J., Majeski, E., & Kudowor, M. (2022). Psychedelic integration: An analysis of the concept and its practice. Frontiers in Psychology.

15. Beck, J. S., & Beck, A. T. (2011). Cognitive behavior therapy: Basics and beyond (2nd ed.). Guilford Press.

16. Beckley Foundation: www.beckleyfoundation.org The Beckley Foundation engages in research and policy work to develop evidence-based drug policies and to investigate the effects of psychoactive substances on the brain and consciousness.

17. Begley, S. (2007). Train your mind, change your brain: How a new science reveals our extraordinary potential to transform ourselves. Ballantine Books.

18. Bennet, H. (2019). Compassion for one's self in PTSD: The role of self-compassion in trauma therapy. Journal of Aggression, Maltreatment & Trauma, 28(6), 714-730.

19. Berman, R. M., Cappiello, A., Anand, A., Oren, D. A., Heninger, G. R., Charney, D. S., & Krystal, J. H. (2000). Antidepressant effects of ketamine in depressed patients. Biological Psychiatry, 47(4), 351-354.

20. Biscoe, N., Bonson, A., Slavin, M., Busuttil, W., et al. (2023). Psilocybin-assisted psychotherapy for the treatment of PTSD in UK armed forces veterans: A feasibility study protocol. European Journal of Psychiatry.

21. Bisson, J. I., Cosgrove, S., Lewis, C., & Robert, N. P. (2015). Post-traumatic stress disorder. BMJ, 351, h6161. doi:10.1136/bmj.h6161

22. Bisson, J. I., Roberts, N. P., Andrew, M., Cooper, R., & Lewis, C. (2013). Psychological therapies for chronic post-traumatic stress disorder (PTSD) in adults. Cochrane Database of Systematic Reviews, 2013(12). doi:10.1002/14651858.CD003388.pub4

23. Boakye, E., et al. (2017). Prevalence of depression among veterans: A systematic review and meta-analysis. Journal of Affective Disorders, 217, 197-204.

24. Bogenschutz, M. P., & Johnson, M. W. (2016). Classic hallucinogens in the treatment of addictions. Progress in Neuro-Psychopharmacology & Biological Psychiatry, 64, 250-258.

25. Bogenschutz, M. P., & Johnson, M. W. (2016). Classic hallucinogens in the treatment of addictions. Progress in Neuro-Psychopharmacology and Biological Psychiatry, 64, 250-258.

26. Bogenschutz, M. P., & Johnson, M. W. (2016). Classic hallucinogens in the treatment of addictions. Progress in Neuro-Psychopharmacology and Biological Psychiatry, 64, 250-258.

27. Bogenschutz, M. P., Forcehimes, A. A., Pommy, J. A., Wilcox, C. E., Barbosa, P. C. R., & Strassman, R. J. (2015). Psilocybin-assisted treatment for alcohol dependence: A proof-of-concept study. Journal of Psychopharmacology, 29(3), 289-299.

28. Bordin, E. S. (1979). The Generalizability of the Psychoanalytic Concept of the Working Alliance. Psychotherapy: Theory, Research & Practice.

29. Botella, C., Serrano, B., Baños, R. M., & Garcia-Palacios, A. (2015). Virtual reality exposure-based therapy for anxiety disorders: A meta-analysis. Journal of Anxiety Disorders, 35, 26-34. doi:10.1016/j.janxdis.2015.08.005

30. Bouso, J. C., Palhano-Fontes, F., Rodríguez-Fornells, A., Ribeiro, S., Sanches, R., Crippa, J. A., ... & Riba, J. (2015). Long-term use of psychedelic drugs is associated with differences in brain structure and personality in humans. European Neuropsychopharmacology, 25(4), 483-492.
31. Bowen, M. (1978). Family therapy in clinical practice. New York: Jason Aronson.
32. Bowlby, J. (1982). Attachment and Loss: Vol. 1. Attachment. Basic Books.
33. Bradberry, T., & Greaves, J. (2009). Emotional Intelligence 2.0. TalentSmart.
34. Bremner, J. D., Southwick, S. M., Darnell, A., & Charney, D. S. (1996). Chronic PTSD in Vietnam combat veterans: Course of illness and substance abuse. The American Journal of Psychiatry, 153(3), 369-375.
35. Brown, G. K., Ten Have, T., Henriques, G. R., Xie, S. X., Hollander, J. E., & Beck, A. T. (2016). Cognitive therapy for the prevention of suicide attempts: A randomized controlled trial. JAMA Psychiatry, 63(8), 801-809. doi:10.1001/jamapsychiatry.2016.1133.
36. Brown, T. K. (2013). Ibogaine in the Treatment of Substance Dependence. Current Drug Abuse Reviews, 6(1), 3-16.
37. Brown, T. K. (2013). Ibogaine in the treatment of substance dependence. Current Drug Abuse Reviews, 6(1), 3-16.
38. Brown, T. K., & Alper, K. R. (2017). Treatment of opioid use disorder with ibogaine: Detoxification and drug use outcomes. The American Journal of Drug and Alcohol Abuse, 43(1), 24-36.
39. Caporuscio, C. (2022). Belief now, true belief later: The epistemic advantage of self-related insights in psychedelic-assisted therapy. Philosophy and the Mind Sciences, 3, 7.
40. Carhart-Harris, R. L., & Friston, K. J. (2019). REBUS and the anarchic brain: Toward a unified model of the brain action of psychedelics. Pharmacological Reviews, 71(3), 316-344.

41. Carhart-Harris, R. L., & Goodwin, G. M. (2017). The therapeutic potential of psychedelic drugs: Past, present, and future. Neuropsychopharmacology, 42(11), 2105-2113.

42. Carhart-Harris, R. L., & Goodwin, G. M. (2017). The therapeutic potential of psychedelic drugs: past, present, and future. Neuropsychopharmacology, 42(11), 2105-2113.

43. Carhart-Harris, R. L., & Nutt, D. J. (2014). Serotonin and brain function: A tale of two receptors. Journal of Psychopharmacology, 28(9), 865-875.

44. Carhart-Harris, R. L., Bolstridge, M., Day, C. M. J., Rucker, J., Watts, R., Erritzoe, D. E., ... & Nutt, D. J. (2018). Psilocybin with psychological support for treatment-resistant depression: An open-label feasibility study. The Lancet Psychiatry, 3(7), 619-627.

45. Carhart-Harris, R. L., et al. (2016). Psilocybin with psychological support for treatment-resistant depression: An open-label feasibility study. The Lancet Psychiatry, 3(7), 619-627.

46. Chambers, R., Stoliker, D., & Simonsson, O. (2023). Psychedelic-Assisted Psychotherapy and Mindfulness-Based Cognitive Therapy: Potential Synergies. Mindfulness.

47. Ciccarelli, S. K., & White, J. N. (2015). Psychology (4th ed.). Pearson.

48. Ciccarelli, S. K., & White, J. N. (2015). Psychology (4th ed.). Upper Saddle River, NJ: Pearson Education.

49. Corcoran, J. (2006). Cognitive-behavioral methods: A workbook for social workers. Allyn & Bacon.

50. Cornish, S., et al. (2014). The rise in mental health diagnoses among US military personnel, veterans, and their families. Military Medicine, 179(8), 902-911.

51. Coursera. (n.d.). The Science of Well-Being. Retrieved from https://www.coursera.org/learn/the-science-of-well-being

52. Cucciare, M. A., Weingardt, K. R., & Humphreys, K. (2016). How Internet technology can improve the quality of care for

substance use disorders. Current Drug Abuse Reviews, 3(3), 256-262. doi:10.2174/1874473711003030256.

53. Currier, J. M., Holland, J. M., & Malott, J. (2015). Moral injury, meaning making, and mental health in returning veterans. Journal of Clinical Psychology, 71(3), 229-240. doi:10.1002/jclp.22134.

54. Davis, A. K., Averill, L. A., Sepeda, N. D., et al. (2020). Psychedelic treatment for trauma-related psychological and cognitive impairment among US special operations forces veterans. Chronic Stress, 4.

55. Davis, A. K., Barrett, F. S., & Griffiths, R. R. (2020). Psychological flexibility mediates the relations between acute psychedelic effects and subjective decreases in depression and anxiety. Journal of Contextual Behavioral Science, 15, 39-45.

56. Davis, A. K., Barrett, F. S., & Griffiths, R. R. (2021). Psychological flexibility mediates the relations between acute psychedelic effects and subjective decreases in depression and anxiety. Journal of Contextual Behavioral Science, 18, 24-31.

57. Davis, A. K., Barsuglia, J. P., Lancelotta, R., Grant, R. M., & Renn, E. (2017). The epidemiology of ibogaine use in the United States. Journal of Psychoactive Drugs, 49(1), 1-10.

58. Davis, A. K., Levin, A. W., Nagib, P. B., Armstrong, S. B., et al. (2023). Study protocol of an open-label proof-of-concept trial examining the safety and clinical efficacy of psilocybin-assisted therapy for veterans with PTSD. BMJ Open, 13(1).

59. Davis, A. K., So, S., Lancelotta, R., Barsuglia, J. P., & Griffiths, R. R. (2019). 5-MeO-DMT administration is associated with subjective improvements in depression and anxiety. The American Journal of Drug and Alcohol Abuse, 45(2), 161-169. DOI: 10.1080/00952990.2018.1545024

60. Davis, A. K., et al. (2020). Veterans' experiences with ayahuasca for the treatment of PTSD: A qualitative analysis. Journal of Psychoactive Drugs, 52(4), 287-294.

61. Doblin, R., Jerome, L., & Anderson, B. T. (2020). The past and future of psychedelic science: An introduction to this issue. Journal of Psychoactive Drugs, 52(1), 1-15.

62. Earleywine, M., Low, F., Lau, C., et al. (2022). Integration in psychedelic-assisted treatments: Recurring themes in current providers' definitions, challenges, and concerns. Journal of Humanistic Psychology.

63. Elbogen, E. B., et al. (2012). Homelessness and suicide risk among veterans: A literature review. Suicide and Life-Threatening Behavior, 42(1), 7-19.

64. Elnitsky, C., et al. (2017). Health and social conditions of homeless veterans: A systematic literature review. Military Behavioral Health, 5(1), 42-55.

65. Espejo, E. P., et al. (2016). Anxiety disorders in veterans: Prevalence, types, and management. Journal of Military and Veterans' Health, 24(4), 44-53.

66. Farb, N. A. S., Anderson, A. K., & Segal, Z. V. (2012). The mindful brain and emotion regulation in mood disorders. Canadian Journal of Psychiatry, 57(2), 70-77. doi:10.1177/070674371205700203.

67. Feder, A., Parides, M. K., Murrough, J. W., Perez, A. M., Morgan, J. E., Saxena, S., ... & Charney, D. S. (2014). Efficacy of intravenous ketamine for treatment of chronic posttraumatic stress disorder: A randomized clinical trial. JAMA Psychiatry, 71(6), 681-688.

68. Feder, A., Parides, M. K., Murrough, J. W., Perez, A. M., Morgan, J. E., Saxena, S., ... & Charney, D. S. (2014). Efficacy of intravenous ketamine for treatment of chronic posttraumatic stress disorder: A randomized clinical trial. JAMA Psychiatry, 71(6), 681-688.

69. Feduccia, A. A., Holland, J., & Mithoefer, M. C. (2018). Progress and promise for the MDMA drug development program. Psychopharmacology, 235(2), 561-571.

70. Feduccia, A. A., Holland, J., & Mithoefer, M. C. (2018). Progress and promise for the MDMA drug development program. Psychopharmacology, 235(2), 561-571.

71. Feduccia, A. A., Jerome, L., Yazar-Klosinski, B., Emerson, A., Mithoefer, M. C., & Doblin, R. (2019). Breakthrough for trauma treatment: Safety and efficacy of MDMA-assisted psychotherapy compared to paroxetine and sertraline. Frontiers in Psychiatry, 10, 650.

72. Ferruolo DM. Psychosocial Equine Program for Veterans. Soc Work. 2016 Jan;61(1):53-60. doi: 10.1093/sw/swv054. PMID: 26897999.

73. Ferruolo, D. (2005). Elements of life success. MountainLake Publishing.

74. Ferruolo, D. (2014). Insights from working with veterans. In J. Marich (Ed.), Trauma made simple (pp. 1-250). Hauppage, NY: Nova.

75. Ferruolo, D. (2014). Insights from working with veterans. In: Marich, J. (2014).

76. Ferruolo, D. (2024). Connecting with the bliss of life. Tattered Press.

77. Ferruolo, D. M. (2016). Psychosocial Equine Program for Veterans. Social Work, 61(1), 53-60. doi:10.1093/sw/swv054

78. Ferruolo, D. M. (2018). Veteran Focused Equine Facilitated Mental Health. ProQuest Dissertations Publishing. (No. 13426630). Plymouth State University.

79. Fiore, L. D. (2014). Cognitive behavioral therapy for anxiety and depression. Veterans Affairs.

80. Frecska, E., Bokor, P., & Winkelman, M. (2016). The therapeutic potentials of ayahuasca: Possible effects against various diseases of civilization. Frontiers in Pharmacology, 7, 35.

81. Frymann, T., Whitney, S., Yaden, D. B., Lipson, J. (2022). The Psychedelic Integration Scales: Tools for Measuring Psychedelic Integration Behaviors and Experiences. Frontiers in Psychology.

82. Garcia, H. A., Kelley, L. P., Rentz, T. O., & Lee, S. (2011). Pretreatment predictors of dropout from cognitive behavioral therapy for PTSD in Iraq and Afghanistan war veterans. Psychological Services, 8(1), 1-11. doi:10.1037/a0022705.

83. Garcia-Romeu, A., Griffiths, R. R., & Johnson, M. W. (2014). Psilocybin-occasioned mystical experiences in the treatment of tobacco addiction. Current Drug Abuse Reviews, 7(3), 157-164.

84. Garcia-Romeu, A., Griffiths, R. R., & Johnson, M. W. (2014). Psilocybin-occasioned mystical experiences in the treatment of tobacco addiction. Current Drug Abuse Reviews, 7(3), 157-164.

85. Garcia-Romeu, A., Kersgaard, B., & Addy, P. H. (2016). Clinical applications of hallucinogens: A review. Experimental and Clinical Psychopharmacology, 24(4), 229-268.

86. Garcia-Romeu, A., Kersgaard, B., & Addy, P. H. (2016). Clinical applications of hallucinogens: A review. Experimental and Clinical Psychopharmacology, 24(4), 229-268.

87. Gasser, P., Holstein, D., Michel, Y., Doblin, R., Yazar-Klosinski, B., Passie, T., & Brenneisen, R. (2014). Safety and efficacy of lysergic acid diethylamide-assisted psychotherapy for anxiety associated with life-threatening diseases. The Journal of Nervous and Mental Disease, 202(7), 513-520.

88. Germer, C. K., Siegel, R. D., & Fulton, P. R. (Eds.). (2013). Mindfulness and psychotherapy (2nd ed.). Guilford Press.

89. Glick, S. D., & Maisonneuve, I. M. (2000). Mechanisms of anti-addictive actions of ibogaine. Annals of the New York Academy of Sciences, 914(1), 394-401.

90. Goleman, D. (1995). Emotional Intelligence: Why It Can Matter More Than IQ. Bantam Books.

91. Gould, C. E., et al. (2016). Anxiety disorders in older veterans: Prevalence and management. Clinical Gerontologist, 39(5), 377-391.

92. Gray, J. C., Murphy, M., Carter, S. E., et al. (2022). Beliefs and Perceived Barriers Regarding Psychedelic-assisted Therapy in a

Pilot Study of Service Members and Veterans With a History of Traumatic Brain Injury. Military Medicine.

93. Greenway, K. T., Garel, N., Jerome, L., et al. (2020). Integrating psychotherapy and psychopharmacology: psychedelic-assisted psychotherapy and other combined treatments. Expert Review of Neurotherapeutics.

94. Greenway, K. T., Garel, N., Jerome, L., et al. (2020). Integrating psychotherapy and psychopharmacology: psychedelic-assisted psychotherapy and other combined treatments. Expert Review of Pharmacoeconomics & Outcomes Research, 20(6).

95. Griffiths, R. R., Johnson, M. W., Carducci, M. A., Umbricht, A., Richards, W. A., Richards, B. D., & Klinedinst, M. A. (2016). Psilocybin produces substantial and sustained decreases in depression and anxiety in patients with life-threatening cancer: A randomized double-blind trial. Journal of Psychopharmacology, 30(12).

96. Griffiths, R. R., Johnson, M. W., Carducci, M. A., Umbricht, A., Richards, W. A., Richards, B. D., ... & Klinedinst, M. A. (2016). Psilocybin produces substantial and sustained decreases in depression and anxiety in patients with life-threatening cancer: A randomized double-blind trial. Journal of Psychopharmacology, 30(12), 1181-1197.

97. Griffiths, R. R., Johnson, M. W., Carducci, M. A., Umbricht, A., Richards, W. A., Richards, B. D., Cosimano, M. P., & Klinedinst, M. A. (2016). Psilocybin produces substantial and sustained decreases in depression and anxiety in patients with life-threatening cancer: A randomized double-blind trial. Journal of Psychopharmacology, 30(12), 1181-1197.

98. Griffiths, R. R., Johnson, M. W., Carducci, M. A., Umbricht, A., Richards, W. A., Richards, B. D., Cosimano, M. P., & Klinedinst, M. A. (2016). Psilocybin produces substantial and sustained decreases in depression and anxiety in patients with life-threatening cancer: A randomized double-blind trial. Journal

of Psychopharmacology, 30(12), 1181-1197. https://doi.org/10.1177/0269881116675513

99. Griffiths, R. R., Johnson, M. W., Richards, W. A., Richards, B. D., McCann, U., & Jesse, R. (2011). Psilocybin occasioned mystical-type experiences: Immediate and persisting dose-related effects. Psychopharmacology, 218(4), 649-665. DOI: 10.1007/s00213-011-2358-5

100. Griffiths, R. R., et al. (2011). Psilocybin occasioned mystical-type experiences: Immediate and persisting dose-related effects. Psychopharmacology, 218(4), 649-665.

101. Grigsby, J., et al. (2021). Psychedelics in the treatment of PTSD: A comprehensive review of evidence, challenges, and future directions. Journal of Traumatic Stress, 34(2), 281-292.

102. Grob, C. S., & Bossis, A. P. (2017). The Psychedelic Renaissance: Reassessing the Role of Psychedelic Drugs in 21st Century Psychiatry and Society. Springer.

103. Grob, C. S., Danforth, A. L., Chopra, G. S., Hagerty, M., McKay, C. R., Halberstadt, A. L., & Greer, G. R. (2011). Pilot study of psilocybin treatment for anxiety in patients with advanced-stage cancer. Archives of General Psychiatry, 68(1), 71-78.

104. Grob, C. S., McKenna, D. J., Callaway, J. C., Brito, G. S., Neves, E. S., Oberlaender, G., ... & Strassman, R. J. (1996). Human psychopharmacology of hoasca, a plant hallucinogen used in ritual context in Brazil. The Journal of Nervous and Mental Disease, 184(2), 86-94.

105. Grof, S. (2000). Psychology of the Future: Lessons from Modern Consciousness Research. State University of New York Press.

106. Grof, S. (2001). LSD Psychotherapy. MAPS. A foundational text on the therapeutic use of LSD, discussing its potential for providing access to the unconscious mind.

107. Grof, S. (2001). LSD Psychotherapy: Exploring the Frontiers of the Hidden Mind. MAPS.

108. Grof, S. (2001). LSD psychotherapy. Ben Lomond, CA: Multidisciplinary Association for Psychedelic Studies.

109. Grof, S., & Halifax, J. (1977). The Human Encounter With Death. E.P. Dutton.

110. Halberstadt, A. L. (2015). Recent advances in the neuropsychopharmacology of serotonergic hallucinogens. Behavioural Brain Research, 277, 99-120.

111. Halpern, J. H., Sherwood, A. R., Passie, T., Blackwell, K. C., & Ruttenber, A. J. (2008). Evidence of health and safety in American members of a religion who use a hallucinogenic sacrament. Medical Science Monitor, 14(8), SR15-SR22.

112. Hartogsohn, I. (2016). Set and setting, psychedelics and the placebo response: An extra-pharmacological perspective on psychopharmacology. Journal of Psychopharmacology, 30(12), 1259-1267.

113. Hartogsohn, I. (2016). Set and setting, psychedelics and the placebo response: An extra-pharmacological perspective on psychopharmacology. Journal of Psychopharmacology, 30(12).

114. Hartogsohn, I. (2017). Constructing drug effects: A history of set and setting. Drug Science, Policy and Law, 3, 1-17.

115. Hasler, G. (2023). Psychotherapy and psychedelic drugs. The Lancet Psychiatry, 10(1).

116. Hawryluk, M., & Ridley-Kerr, R. (2012). Veteran homelessness: A supplementary report to the 2012 annual homeless assessment report. Washington, DC: U.S. Department of Housing and Urban Development.

117. Heffter Research Institute: www.heffter.org This institute supports research into the therapeutic uses of psilocybin and other psychedelics, with a focus on alleviating suffering and improving the quality of life.

118. Hoener, S., Wolfgang, A., Nissan, D., & Howe, E. (2023). Ethical considerations for psychedelic-assisted therapy in military clinical settings. Journal of Medical Ethics.

119. Hoffman, R., Ruck, C., & Staples, B. D. (2008). The hidden world in Homer's Odyssey: A discovery of shamanic trance-

inducing plants and substances. Journal of Ethnopharmacology, 115(2), 152-160.

120. Hofmann, A. (1980). The Mexican relatives of LSD. Journal of Psychedelic Drugs, 12(1), 41-43.

121. Hofmann, A., & Schultes, R. E. (1979). Plants of the gods: Origins of hallucinogenic use. New York: McGraw-Hill.

122. Hoge, C. W., et al. (2004). Combat duty in Iraq and Afghanistan, mental health problems, and barriers to care. New England Journal of Medicine, 351(1), 13-22.

123. Holmes, J. (2002). John Bowlby and attachment theory. Routledge.

124. Hooyer, K., Applbaum, K., et al. (2020). Altered states of combat: Veteran trauma and the quest for novel therapeutics in psychedelic substances. Journal of Humanistic Psychology, 61(3).

125. Howell, E., & Wool, Z. H. (2011). A critical approach to homelessness among veterans in the US. American Journal of Public Health, 101(S1), S236-S237.

126. Huxley, A. (1954). The Doors of Perception. Harper & Brothers.

127. Huxley, A. (1990). The Doors of Perception and Heaven and Hell. Harper & Row.

128. James, W. (1902). The varieties of religious experience: A study in human nature. New York, NY: Longmans, Green & Co.

129. Jay, M. (2019). Mescaline: A Global History of the First Psychedelic. Yale University Press.

130. Jay, M. (2019). Mescaline: A global history of the first psychedelic. Yale University Press.

131. Johnson, M. W., Garcia-Romeu, A., & Griffiths, R. R. (2017). Long-term follow-up of psilocybin-assisted psychotherapy for psychiatric and existential distress in patients with life-threatening cancer. Journal of Psychopharmacology, 31(2), 116-134.

132. Johnson, M. W., Garcia-Romeu, A., & Griffiths, R. R. (2017). Long-term follow-up of psilocybin-facilitated smoking cessation. The American Journal of Drug and Alcohol Abuse, 43(1), 55-60.

133. Johnson, M. W., Garcia-Romeu, A., Cosimano, M. P., & Griffiths, R. R. (2014). Pilot study of the 5-HT2AR agonist psilocybin in the treatment of tobacco addiction. Journal of Psychopharmacology, 28(11), 983-992.

134. Johnson, M. W., Richards, W. A., & Griffiths, R. R. (2008). Human hallucinogen research: Guidelines for safety. Journal of Psychopharmacology, 22(6), 603-620.

135. Johnson, M. W., et al. (2019). Pilot study of the 5-HT2AR agonist psilocybin in the treatment of tobacco addiction. Journal of Psychopharmacology, 28(11), 983-992.

136. Jung, C. G. (1953). Two essays on analytical psychology (Collected Works of C.G. Jung, Volume 7). Princeton, NJ: Princeton University Press.

137. Kabat-Zinn, J. (2013). Full catastrophe living: Using the wisdom of your body and mind to face stress, pain, and illness (Revised ed.). Bantam Books.

138. Kaplan, J. B., Bergman, A. L., Christopher, M., Bowen, S., & Hunsinger, M. (2012). Role of resilience in mindfulness training for first responders. Mindfulness, 3(4), 291-301. doi:10.1007/s12671-012-0103-0

139. Kaplan, M. S., et al. (2012). Suicide among male veterans: A prospective population-based study. Journal of Epidemiology and Community Health, 66(7), 622-627.

140. Karstoft, K. I., Nielsen, A. B., & Nielsen, A. S. (2017). Depression among returning veterans: A longitudinal analysis. Journal of Affective Disorders, 210, 312-318.

141. Keane, T. M., Marshall, A. D., & Taft, C. T. (2006). Posttraumatic stress disorder: Etiology, epidemiology, and treatment outcome. Annual Review of Clinical Psychology, 2, 161-197. doi:10.1146/annurev.clinpsy.2.022305.095305

142. Kehle-Forbes, S. M., Meis, L. A., Spoont, M. R., & Polusny, M. A. (2016). Treatment Engagement and Response to CBT among Veterans with PTSD. Journal of Consulting and Clinical Psychology.

143. Kopacz, M. S., & Connery, A. L. (2015). The veterans affairs moral injury workgroup: Recommendations and priorities. Journal of Rehabilitation Research & Development, 52(5), vii-x.

144. Krippner, S., & Welch, P. (1992). Spiritual dimensions of healing: From native shamanism to contemporary health care. New York: Irvington.

145. Krystal, J. H., & Neumeister, A. (2009). Noradrenergic and serotonergic mechanisms in the neurobiology of posttraumatic stress disorder and resilience. Brain Research, 1293, 13-23. doi:10.1016/j.brainres.2009.03.044

146. Krystal, J. H., Abdallah, C. G., Averill, L. A., Kelmendi, B., Harpaz-Rotem, I., Sanacora, G., ... & D'Souza, D. C. (2020). Synaptic loss and the pathophysiology of PTSD: Implications for ketamine as a prototype novel therapeutic. Current Psychiatry Reports, 22(10), 61.

147. Krystal, J. H., Abdallah, C. G., Sanacora, G., Charney, D. S., & Duman, R. S. (2019). Ketamine: A Paradigm Shift for Depression Research and Treatment. Neuron, 101(5), 774-778.

148. Krystal, J. H., Abdallah, C. G., Sanacora, G., Charney, D. S., & Duman, R. S. (2019). Ketamine: A paradigm shift for depression research and treatment. Neuron, 101(5), 774-778.

149. Krystal, J. H., Abdallah, C. G., Sanacora, G., Charney, D. S., & Duman, R. S. (2019). Ketamine: A paradigm shift for depression research and treatment. Neuron, 101(5), 774-778.

150. Krystal, J. H., Karper, L. P., Seibyl, J. P., Freeman, G. K., Delaney, R., Bremner, J. D., ... & Charney, D. S. (1994). Subanesthetic effects of the noncompetitive NMDA antagonist, ketamine, in humans: Psychotomimetic, perceptual, cognitive, and neuroendocrine responses. Archives of General Psychiatry, 51(3), 199-214.

151. LaBarre, W. (1975). The peyote cult (Vol. 10). Yale University Press.

152. LaBarre, W. (1975). The peyote cult. Yale University Press.

153. Labate, B. C., & Cavnar, C. (2014). The therapeutic use of Ayahuasca. Springer.

154. Labate, B. C., & Cavnar, C. (Eds.). (2014). Ayahuasca shamanism in the Amazon and beyond. Oxford University Press.

155. Leary, T., Litwin, G. H., & Metzner, R. (1963). Reactions to psilocybin administered in a supportive environment. The Journal of Nervous and Mental Disease, 137(6), 561-573.

156. Litz, B. T., Stein, N., Delaney, E., Lebowitz, L., Nash, W. P., Silva, C., & Maguen, S. (2009). Moral injury and moral repair in war veterans: A preliminary model and intervention strategy. Clinical Psychology Review, 29(8), 695-706.

157. Litz, B. T., et al. (2009). Moral injury and moral repair in war veterans: A preliminary model and intervention strategy. Clinical Psychology Review, 29(8), 695-706.

158. Lotsof, H. S., & Alexander, N. E. (2001). Case studies of ibogaine treatment: Implications for patient management strategies. Alkaloids: Chemical and Biological Perspectives, 56, 293-313.

159. Luoma, J. B., Chwyl, C., Bathje, G. J., Davis, A. K., et al. (2020). A meta-analysis of placebo-controlled trials of psychedelic-assisted therapy. Journal of Contextual Behavioral Science, 17, 41-59.

160. Luoma, J. B., Sabucedo, P., Eriksson, J., Gates, N., et al. (2019). Toward a contextual psychedelic-assisted therapy: perspectives from acceptance and commitment therapy and contextual behavioral science. Journal of Contextual Behavioral Science, 12, 109-117.

161. Lutz, P. E., & Kieffer, B. L. (2013). Opioid receptors: Distinct roles in mood disorders. Trends in Neurosciences, 36(3), 195-206.

162. MAPS (Multidisciplinary Association for Psychedelic Studies). (n.d.). Research on MDMA-assisted Psychotherapy.

163. MAPS - Multidisciplinary Association for Psychedelic Studies. (n.d.). Retrieved from https://maps.org/

164. MAPS Public Benefit Corporation. (2021). MDMA-assisted psychotherapy. Multidisciplinary Association for Psychedelic Studies (MAPS) Public Benefit Corporation (MAPS PBC).

165. Mabit, J., Giove, R., & Vega, J. (1996). Takiwasi: The use of Amazonian shamanism to rehabilitate drug addicts. In C. S. Grob (Ed.), Hallucinogens: A reader (pp. 87-105). Tarcher/Putnam.

166. MacLean, K. A., Johnson, M. W., & Griffiths, R. R. (2011). Mystical experiences occasioned by the hallucinogen psilocybin lead to increases in the personality domain of openness. Journal of Psychopharmacology, 25(11), 1453-1461.

167. MacLean, K. A., Johnson, M. W., & Griffiths, R. R. (2011). Mystical experiences occasioned by the hallucinogen psilocybin lead to increases in the personality domain of openness. Journal of Psychopharmacology, 25(11), 1453-1461. https://doi.org/10.1177/0269881111420188

168. MacLean, K. A., Johnson, M. W., & Griffiths, R. R. (2011). Mystical experiences occasioned by the hallucinogen psilocybin lead to increases in the personality domain of openness. Journal of Psychopharmacology, 25(11).

169. Macias, C., Barreira, P., Alden, M., & Boyd, J. W. (2016). The ICCD clubhouse model: Mental health rehabilitation and recovery. Psychiatric Services, 67(5), 476-482. doi:10.1176/appi.ps.201400529

170. Mash, D. C., & Kovera, C. A. (1999). Ibogaine: Complex pharmacokinetics, concerns for safety, and preliminary efficacy measures. Annals of the New York Academy of Sciences, 844(1), 358-360.

171. Mash, D. C., Kovera, C. A., Buck, B. E., Norenberg, M. D., Shapshak, P., Hearn, W. L., & Sanchez-Ramos, J. (1998). Medication Development of Ibogaine as a Pharmacotherapy for Drug Dependence. Annals of the New York Academy of Sciences, 844(1), 274-292.

172. Maté, G. (2008). In the realm of hungry ghosts: Close encounters with addiction. Berkeley, CA: North Atlantic Books.

173. MentalHealth.va.gov - U.S. Department of Veterans Affairs. (n.d.). Mental Health. Retrieved from https://www.mental-health.va.gov/

174. Metzner, R. (2005). Ayahuasca: Hallucinogens, Consciousness, and the Spirit of Nature. Thunder's Mouth Press.

175. Metzner, R. (2005). Sacred vine of spirits: Ayahuasca. Park Street Press.

176. Minuchin, S. (1974). Families and Family Therapy. Harvard University Press.

177. Mitchell, J. M., Bogenschutz, M., Lilienstein, A., Harrison, C., Kleiman, S., Parker-Guilbert, K., ... & Doblin, R. (2021). MDMA-assisted therapy for severe PTSD: A randomized, double-blind, placebo-controlled phase 3 study. Nature Medicine, 27(6), 1025-1033.

178. Mitchell, J. M., Bogenschutz, M., Lilienstein, A., et al. (2021). MDMA-assisted therapy for severe PTSD: a randomized, double-blind, placebo-controlled phase 3 study. Nature Medicine, 27(6).

179. Mithoefer, M. C., Grob, C. S., & Brewerton, T. D. (2016). Novel psychopharmacological therapies for psychiatric disorders: Psilocybin and MDMA. The Lancet Psychiatry, 3(5), 481-488.

180. Mithoefer, M. C., Jerome, L., & Doblin, R. (2019). MDMA-assisted psychotherapy for posttraumatic stress disorder: A review of the literature and preliminary clinical results from ongoing trials. Journal of Psychoactive Drugs, 51(2), 127-138.

181. Mithoefer, M. C., Mithoefer, A. T., Feduccia, A. A., Jerome, L., Wagner, M., Wymer, J., ... & Doblin, R. (2018). 3,4-methylenedioxymethamphetamine (MDMA)-assisted psychotherapy for post-traumatic stress disorder in military veterans, firefighters, and police officers: A randomised, double-blind, dose-response, phase 2 clinical trial. The Lancet Psychiatry, 5(6), 486-497

182. Mithoefer, M. C., Mithoefer, A. T., Feduccia, A. A., Jerome, L., Wagner, M., Wymer, J., ... & Doblin, R. (2018). 3,4-methylenedioxymethamphetamine (MDMA)-assisted psychotherapy for post-traumatic stress disorder in military veterans, firefighters, and police officers: A randomised, double-blind, dose-response, phase 2 clinical trial. The Lancet Psychiatry, 5(6), 486-497.

183. Mithoefer, M. C., Mithoefer, A. T., Feduccia, A. A., Jerome, L., Wagner, M., Wymer, J., ... & Doblin, R. (2018). 3,4-methylenedioxymethamphetamine (MDMA)-assisted psychotherapy for post-traumatic stress disorder in military veterans, firefighters, and police officers: a randomized, double-blind, dose-response, phase 2 clinical trial. The Lancet Psychiatry, 5(6), 486-497.

184. Mithoefer, M. C., Mithoefer, A. T., Feduccia, A. A., Jerome, L., Wagner, M., Wymer, J., Holland, J., Hamilton, S., Yazar-Klosinski, B., Emerson, A., & Doblin, R. (2019). 3,4-methylenedioxymethamphetamine (MDMA)-assisted psychotherapy for post-traumatic stress disorder in military veterans, firefighters, and police officers: A randomised, double-blind, dose-response, phase 2 clinical trial. The Lancet Psychiatry, 5(6), 486-497.

185. Mithoefer, M. C., Wagner, M. T., Mithoefer, A. T., Jerome, L., & Doblin, R. (2011). The safety and efficacy of ±3, 4-methylenedioxymethamphetamine-assisted psychotherapy in subjects with chronic, treatment-resistant posttraumatic stress disorder: The first randomized controlled pilot study. Journal of Psychopharmacology, 25(4), 439-452.

186. Mithoefer, M. C., Wagner, M. T., Mithoefer, A. T., Jerome, L., & Doblin, R. (2011). The safety and efficacy of ±3,4-methylenedioxymethamphetamine-assisted psychotherapy in subjects with chronic, treatment-resistant posttraumatic stress disorder: The first randomized controlled pilot study. Journal of Psychopharmacology, 25(4), 439-452.

187. Mithoefer, M. C., Wagner, M. T., Mithoefer, A. T., Jerome, L., & Doblin, R. (2011). The safety and efficacy of ±3,4-methylenedioxymethamphetamine-assisted psychotherapy in subjects with chronic, treatment-resistant posttraumatic stress disorder: The first randomized controlled pilot study. Journal of Psychopharmacology, 25(4), 439-452.

188. Mithoefer, M. C., Wagner, M. T., Mithoefer, A. T., Jerome, L., & Doblin, R. (2011). The safety and efficacy of ±3,4-methylenedioxymethamphetamine-assisted psychotherapy in subjects with

chronic, treatment-resistant posttraumatic stress disorder: The first randomized controlled pilot study. Journal of Psychopharmacology, 25(4), 439-452. doi:10.1177/0269881110378371

189. Mithoefer, M. C., Wagner, M. T., Mithoefer, A. T., Jerome, L., & Doblin, R. (2011). The safety and efficacy of ±3,4-methylenedioxymethamphetamine-assisted psychotherapy in subjects with chronic, treatment-resistant posttraumatic stress disorder: the first randomized controlled pilot study. Journal of Psychopharmacology, 25(4), 439-452.

190. Mithoefer, M. C., Wagner, M. T., Mithoefer, A. T., Jerome, L., Martin, S. F., Yazar-Klosinski, B., ... & Doblin, R. (2013). Durability of improvement in post-traumatic stress disorder symptoms and absence of harmful effects or drug dependency after 3,4-methylenedioxymethamphetamine-assisted psychotherapy: A prospective long-term follow-up study. Journal of Psychopharmacology, 27(1), 28-39.

191. Mithoefer, M. C., et al. (2018). MDMA-assisted therapy for treatment of PTSD: Study design and rationale for phase 3 trials based on pooled analysis of six phase 2 randomized controlled trials. Psychopharmacology, 235(11), 3255-3275.

192. Monson, C. M., Fredman, S. J., & Adair, K. C. (2011). Cognitive-Behavioral Conjoint Therapy for PTSD: Harnessing the Healing Power of Relationships. Journal of Family Psychology.

193. Montgomery, A. E., et al. (2015). Distinct subpopulations of veterans among the homeless in the U.S. Community Mental Health Journal, 51(7), 765-774.

194. Moore, B. A., & Penk, W. E. (Eds.). (2011). Treating PTSD in military personnel: A clinical handbook. New York, NY: Guilford Press.

195. Multidisciplinary Association for Psychedelic Studies (MAPS): www.maps.org MAPS is a leading organization in psychedelic research, providing information on ongoing studies, educational resources, and advocacy for therapeutic psychedelics.

196. Najavits, L. M. (2002). Seeking safety: A treatment manual for PTSD and substance abuse. New York, NY: Guilford Press.

197. National Coalition for Homeless Veterans. (n.d.). Veteran homelessness. Retrieved from https://nchv.org/veteran-homelessness/

198. Newport, D. J., Carpenter, L. L., McDonald, W. M., Potash, J. B., Tohen, M., Nemeroff, C. B., & APA Council of Research Task Force on Novel Biomarkers and Treatments. (2015). Ketamine and Other NMDA Antagonists: Early Clinical Trials and Possible Mechanisms in Depression. The American Journal of Psychiatry, 172(10), 950-966.

199. Nichols, D. E. (2016). Psychedelics. Pharmacological Reviews, 68(2), 264-355.

200. Nichols, D. E. (2016). Psychedelics. Pharmacological Reviews, 68(2), 264-355.

201. Nichols, D. E. (2016). Psychedelics. Pharmacological Reviews, 68(2), 264-355. DOI: 10.1124/pr.115.011478

202. Nichols, D. E., & Johnson, M. W. (2019). Psychedelics as medicines: An emerging new paradigm. Clinical Pharmacology & Therapeutics, 107(5), 935-937.

203. Nichols, M. P., & Schwartz, R. C. (2006). Family Therapy: Concepts and Methods. Pearson/Allyn & Bacon.

204. Nicholson, H. L., & Balster, R. L. (2021). Psychedelics as a novel approach to treating autoimmune conditions. Immunology Letters, 228.

205. Norcross, J. C., & Lambert, M. J. (2011). Psychotherapy Relationships That Work: Evidence-Based Responsiveness. Oxford University Press.

206. Nutt, D. J., King, L. A., & Nichols, D. E. (2013). Effects of Schedule I drug laws on neuroscience research and treatment innovation. Nature Reviews Neuroscience, 14(8), 577-585.

207. Oehen, P., Traber, R., Widmer, V., & Schnyder, U. (2013). A randomized, controlled pilot study of MDMA (±3,4-Methylene-dioxymethamphetamine)-assisted psychotherapy for treatment

of resistant, chronic Post-Traumatic Stress Disorder (PTSD). Journal of Psychopharmacology, 27(1), 40-52.

208. Oehen, P., Traber, R., Widmer, V., & Schnyder, U. (2013). A randomized, controlled pilot study of MDMA (±3,4-methylenedioxymethamphetamine)-assisted psychotherapy for treatment of resistant, chronic post-traumatic stress disorder (PTSD). Journal of Psychopharmacology, 27(1), 40-52.

209. Olson, D. E. (2021). Psychoplastogens: a promising class of plasticity-promoting neurotherapeutics. Journal of Experimental Neuroscience, 15.

210. Ot'alora G, Grigsby, J., Poulter, B., Van Derveer, J. W., III, Giron, S. G., Jerome, L., ... & Mithoefer, M. C. (2018). 3,4-Methylenedioxymethamphetamine-assisted psychotherapy for treatment of chronic posttraumatic stress disorder: A randomized phase 2 controlled trial. Journal of Psychopharmacology, 32(12), 1295-1307.

211. Ot'alora G, M., Grigsby, J., Poulter, B., Van Derveer, J. W., Giron, S. G., Jerome, L., ... & Mithoefer, M. C. (2018). 3,4-methylenedioxymethamphetamine-assisted psychotherapy for posttraumatic stress disorder in military veterans, firefighters, and police officers: A randomised, double-blind, dose-response, phase 2 clinical trial. The Lancet Psychiatry, 5(6), 486-497.

212. Ozer, E. J., Best, S. R., Lipsey, T. L., & Weiss, D. S. (2003). Predictors of posttraumatic stress disorder and symptoms in adults: A meta-analysis. Psychological Bulletin, 129(1), 52-73. doi:10.1037/0033-2909.129.1.52

213. Pahnke, W. N., Kurland, A. A., Unger, S., Savage, C., & Grof, S. (1970). The experimental use of psychedelic (LSD) psychotherapy. JAMA, 212(11), 1856-1863.

214. Parrott, A. C. (2013). Human psychobiology of MDMA or 'Ecstasy': An overview of 25 years of empirical research. Human Psychopharmacology: Clinical and Experimental, 28(4), 289-307.

215. Pollan, M. (2018). How to Change Your Mind: What the New Science of Psychedelics Teaches Us About Consciousness, Dying, Addiction, Depression, and Transcendence. Penguin Books.

216. Pollan, M. (2018). How to Change Your Mind: What the New Science of Psychedelics Teaches Us About Consciousness, Dying, Addiction, Depression, and Transcendence. Penguin Press.

217. Pollan, M. (2018). How to Change Your Mind: What the New Science of Psychedelics Teaches Us About Consciousness, Dying, Addiction, Depression, and Transcendence. Penguin Press. This book offers an in-depth look at the history and resurgence of research into psychedelic drugs.

218. Pollan, M. (2018). How to change your mind: What the new science of psychedelics teaches us about consciousness, dying, addiction, depression, and transcendence. New York, NY: Penguin Press.

219. Pollan, M. (2018). How to change your mind: What the new science of psychedelics teaches us about consciousness, dying, addiction, depression, and transcendence. New York: Penguin Press.

220. Pollan, M. (2018). How to change your mind: What the new science of psychedelics teaches us about consciousness, dying, addiction, depression, and transcendence. Penguin Books.

221. Rasmussen, K. G., Kung, S., & Lapid, M. I. (2019). Intravenous ketamine for posttraumatic stress disorder: Emerging evidence and open questions. The Journal of Clinical Psychiatry, 80(4), 18r12515.

222. Reiff, C. M., Richman, E. E., Nemeroff, C. B., et al. (2020). Psychedelics and psychedelic-assisted psychotherapy. American Journal of Psychiatry, 177(5), 391-410.

223. Reis, H. T., & Shaver, P. (1988). Intimacy as an Interpersonal Process. Handbook of Personal Relationships.

224. Ricard, M. (2015). Altruism: The power of compassion to change yourself and the world. New York, NY: Little, Brown and Company.

225. Rose, J., & Raine-Smith, H. (2023). EMDR as a preparation and integration tool in psychedelic-assisted therapy: a collaborative case study. Journal of EMDR Practice and Research.

226. Rosen, G. M., & Davison, G. C. (2003). Psychology should list empirically supported principles of change (ESPs) and not credential trademarked therapies or other treatment packages. Behavior Modification, 27(3), 300-312. doi:10.1177/0145445503027003001

227. Rosenberg, M. B. (2003). Nonviolent Communication: A Language of Life. PuddleDancer Press.

228. Ross, S. (2012). Serotonergic hallucinogens and emerging targets for addiction pharmacotherapies. Psychiatric Clinics of North America, 35(2), 357-374. https://doi.org/10.1016/j.psc.2012.04.004

229. Ross, S., Bossis, A., Guss, J., Agin-Liebes, G., Malone, T., Cohen, B., ... & Schmidt, B. L. (2016). Rapid and sustained symptom reduction following psilocybin treatment for anxiety and depression in patients with life-threatening cancer: A randomized controlled trial. Journal of Psychopharmacology, 30(12), 1165-1180.

230. Ross, S., Bossis, A., Guss, J., Agin-Liebes, G., Malone, T., Cohen, B., ... & Schmidt, B. L. (2016). Rapid and sustained symptom reduction following psilocybin treatment for anxiety and depression in patients with life-threatening cancer: A randomized controlled trial. Journal of Psychopharmacology, 30(12), 1165-1180.

231. Ross, S., Bossis, A., Guss, J., Agin-Liebes, G., Malone, T., Cohen, B., ... & Su, Z. (2016). Rapid and sustained symptom reduction following psilocybin treatment for anxiety and depression in patients with life-threatening cancer: A randomized controlled trial. Journal of Psychopharmacology, 30(12), 1165-1180.

232. Ross, S., Bossis, A., Guss, J., Agin-Liebes, G., Malone, T., Cohen, B., ... & Su, Z. (2016). Rapid and sustained symptom reduction following psilocybin treatment for anxiety and depression in patients with life-threatening cancer: a randomized controlled trial. Journal of Psychopharmacology, 30(12), 1165-1180.

233. Rottenberg, J., & Johnson, S. L. (2014). Emotion and psychopathology: Bridging affective and clinical science. American Psychological Association.

234. Rucker, J. J. H., Iliff, J., & Nutt, D. J. (2018). Psychiatry & the psychedelic drugs. Past, present & future. Neuropharmacology, 142.

235. Rätsch, C. (2005). The encyclopedia of psychoactive plants: Ethnopharmacology and its applications. Park Street Press.

236. Scaer, R. C. (2005). The trauma spectrum: Hidden wounds and human resiliency. New York: W. W. Norton & Company.

237. Schaefer, S. B. (2017). The cultural significance of entheogenic substances: The case of the Greek kykeon. Ethnopharmacologic Search for Psychoactive Drugs, 18, 131-138.

238. Schaefer, S. B. (2019). Sacred plants and the cultivation of power in the ancient Andes: Traces of psychoactive alkaloids in archaeological contexts. Journal of Ethnopharmacology, 241, 111982.

239. Schaefer, S. B., Michael, T., & Weil, Z. M. (2019). Psychotherapeutic benefits of psychedelic drugs in combat veterans with post-traumatic stress disorder: A systematic review. Journal of Psychopharmacology, 33(9), 1077-1083.

240. Schenberg, E. E. (2018). Psychedelic-Assisted Psychotherapy: A Paradigm Shift in Psychiatric Research and Development. Frontiers in Pharmacology, 9, 733.

241. Schenberg, E. E., Alexandre, J. F. M., Filev, R., Cravo, A. M., Sato, J. R., Muthukumaraswamy, S. D., ... & Lobão-Soares, B. (2021). Acute psychotropic effects of ayahuasca in indigenous patients with post-traumatic stress disorder. Journal of Clinical Psychopharmacology, 41(4), 376-386.

242. Schmid, Y., Enzler, F., Gasser, P., Grouzmann, E., Preller, K. H., Vollenweider, F. X., & Brenneisen, R. (2015). Acute effects of lysergic acid diethylamide in healthy subjects. Biological Psychiatry, 78(8), 544-553.

243. Sessa, B. (2012). Psychedelic drug treatments: Assisting the therapeutic process. Mental Health Review Journal, 17(1), 51-63.

244. Sessa, B. (2012). The Psychedelic Renaissance: Reassessing the Role of Psychedelic Drugs in 21st Century Psychiatry and Society. Muswell Hill Press. Sessa examines the medical potential

of psychedelics and the growing acceptance of their use in psychiatry.

245. Sessa, B. (2017). MDMA and PTSD treatment: "PTSD: From novel pathophysiology to innovative therapeutics." Neurosci Lett, 649, 176-180.

246. Sessa, B., & Johnson, M. W. (2015). Can psychedelics cure? The British Journal of Psychiatry, 206(4), 282-283. https://doi.org/10.1192/bjp.bp.114.152751

247. Shanon, B. (2002). The Antipodes of the Mind: Charting the Phenomenology of the Ayahuasca Experience. Oxford University Press.

248. Shapiro, F. (2018). Eye movement desensitization and reprocessing (EMDR) therapy: Basic principles, protocols, and procedures (3rd ed.). Guilford Press.

249. Shay, J. (1994). Achilles in Vietnam: Combat trauma and the undoing of character. New York, NY: Atheneum.

250. Shishkova, Y., Khlghatyan, J., & Saghatelyan, A. (2022). The enigmatic mechanism of the psychedelic-induced plasticity. Brain Research Bulletin, 176.

251. Shulgin, A., & Shulgin, A. (1991). PIHKAL: A Chemical Love Story. Transform Press.

252. Shulgin, A., & Shulgin, A. (1991). PIHKAL: A chemical love story. Berkeley, CA: Transform Press.

253. Shulgin, A., & Shulgin, A. (1991). PiHKAL: A Chemical Love Story. Transform Press. While not exclusively about therapy, this book provides insight into the chemistry and effects of phenethylamines, authored by a renowned chemist.

254. Shulgin, A., & Shulgin, A. (1997). TIHKAL: The Continuation. Transform Press.

255. Siegel, D. J. (2010). Mindsight: The new science of personal transformation. New York: Bantam Books.

256. Sienkiewicz, M. M., Galletly, D. C., & Rosenthal, N. E. (2023). The effects of psychedelics on the brain's functional architecture: a review. Psychopharmacology.

257. Smelson, D. A., et al. (2017). Homeless veterans: Perspectives on social services use. Veterans Affairs Policy Analysis, 15(3), 123-137.

258. Steenkamp, M. M., Litz, B. T., Hoge, C. W., & Marmar, C. R. (2015). Psychotherapy for military-related PTSD: A review of randomized clinical trials. JAMA, 314(5), 489-500. doi:10.1001/jama.2015.8370

259. Strassman, R. (1995). Hallucinogenic drugs in psychiatric research and treatment. Perspectives and prospects. The Journal of Nervous and Mental Disease, 183(3), 127-138.

260. Strassman, R. (2000). DMT: The Spirit Molecule. Park Street Press. The book recounts Strassman's research on DMT, including its potential therapeutic effects.

261. Strassman, R. (2001). DMT: The spirit molecule: A doctor's revolutionary research into the biology of near-death and mystical experiences. Park Street Press.

262. Studerus, E., Kometer, M., Hasler, F., & Vollenweider, F. X. (2011). Acute, subacute and long-term subjective effects of psilocybin in healthy humans: A pooled analysis of experimental studies. Journal of Psychopharmacology, 25(11), 1434-1452.

263. Suzuki, D. T. (1956). Zen Buddhism: Selected writings of D.T. Suzuki. New York, NY: Doubleday Anchor Books.

264. Thal, S. B., & Lommen, M. J. (2020). Current perspective on MDMA-assisted psychotherapy for posttraumatic stress disorder. Journal of Contemporary Psychotherapy, 50(1).

265. Thal, S. B., & Lommen, M. J. J. (2018). Current perspective on MDMA-assisted psychotherapy for posttraumatic stress disorder. Journal of Contemporary Psychotherapy, 48(2), 99-108.

266. The Council on Spiritual Practices (CSP): www.csp.org CSP focuses on the spiritual aspects of psychedelic experiences and their therapeutic applications.

267. The Psychedelic Science Funders Collaborative (PSFC): www.psychedelicscience.org PSFC is a community of philanthropists dedicated to supporting psychedelic research and clinical trials.

268. Trauma made simple. Hauppage, NY: Nova.

269. Tupper, K. W. (2015). Psychedelics, dissociation, and meditation: A review of the historical, scientific, and cultural context. Journal of Transpersonal Psychology, 47(1), 19-46.

270. U.S. Census Bureau. (n.d.). American Community Survey. Retrieved from https://www.census.gov/programs-surveys/acs/

271. U.S. Department of Veterans Affairs. (2015). Substance use in veterans. Washington, DC: Author.

272. Uthaug, M. V., Lancelotta, R., van Oorsouw, K., Kuypers, K. P. C., Mason, N., Rak, J., ... & Ramaekers, J. G. (2018). A single inhalation of vapor from dried toad secretion containing 5-methoxy-N,N-dimethyltryptamine (5-MeO-DMT) in a naturalistic setting is related to sustained enhancement of satisfaction with life, mindfulness-related capacities, and a decrement of psychopathological symptoms. Psychopharmacology, 235(9), 2423-2431.

273. Valdez-Bevan, R. (2023). Managing Existential Distress With Post-Psychedelic-Assisted Psychotherapy Group Integration. ProQuest Dissertations Publishing.

274. Van der Kolk, B. A. (2014). The body keeps the score: Brain, mind, and body in the healing of trauma. New York: Viking.

275. Van der Kolk, B. A. (2015). The body keeps the score: Brain, mind, and body in the healing of trauma. Viking.

276. Veterans Affairs Canada. (n.d.). Mental health and wellness.

277. Vollenweider, F. X., & Kometer, M. (2010). The neurobiology of psychedelic drugs: Implications for the treatment of mood disorders. Nature Reviews Neuroscience, 11(9), 642-651.

278. Vollenweider, F. X., & Preller, K. H. (2020). Psychedelic drugs: Neurobiology and potential for treatment of psychiatric disorders. Nature Reviews Neuroscience, 21(11), 611-624.

279. Vujanovic, A. A., Youngwirth, N. E., Johnson, K. A., & Zvolensky, M. J. (2009). Mindfulness-based stress reduction for PTSD among veterans: Preliminary results of a randomized

controlled trial. Journal of Clinical Psychology, 65(7), 881-890. doi:10.1002/jclp.20579

280. Wagner, A. C., Mithoefer, M. C., Daughters, S. B., Doblin, R., & Badour, C. L. (2019). In search of MDMA's fear-extinguishing effects: A systematic review. Frontiers in Psychiatry, 10, 456.

281. Walser, R. D., & Westrup, D. (2007). Acceptance & commitment therapy for the treatment of post-traumatic stress disorder and trauma-related problems: A practitioner's guide to using mindfulness & acceptance strategies. New Harbinger Publications.

282. Walsh, R., & Grob, C. S. (Eds.). (2005). Higher wisdom: Eminent elders explore the continuing impact of psychedelics. Albany, NY: State University of New York Press.

283. Walsh, Z., & Thiessen, M. S. (2018). Psychedelics and the new behaviorism: considering the integration of third-wave behavior therapies with psychedelic-assisted therapy. International Review of Psychiatry, 30(4), 343-349.

284. Waltz, T. J., et al. (2014). Mental health treatment preferences of primary care patients. Journal of Primary Care & Community Health, 5(4), 278-283.

285. Watts, A. (1968). Psychedelics and religious experience. California Law Review, 56(1), 74-85.

286. Watts, A. (2012). Psychotherapy East & West. New World Library.

287. Watts, R., Day, C., Krzanowski, J., Nutt, D., & Carhart-Harris, R. (2017). Patients' accounts of increased "connectedness" and "acceptance" after psilocybin for treatment-resistant depression. Journal of Humanistic Psychology, 57(5), 520-564.

288. Wheeler, S. W., & Dyer, N. L. (2020). A systematic review of psychedelic-assisted psychotherapy for mental health: An evaluation of the current wave of research and suggestions for the future. Psychology of Consciousness: Theory, Research, and Practice, 7(1), 59-70.

289. Wilkinson, S. T., Ballard, E. D., Bloch, M. H., Mathew, S. J., Murrough, J. W., Feder, A., ... & Sanacora, G. (2018). The effect of a single dose of intravenous ketamine on suicidal ideation: A

systematic review and individual participant data meta-analysis. American Journal of Psychiatry, 175(2), 150-158.

290. Winkelman, M. (2014). Psychedelics as medicines for substance abuse rehabilitation: Evaluating treatments with LSD, Peyote, Ibogaine and Ayahuasca. Current Drug Abuse Reviews, 7(2), 101-116.

291. Winkelman, M., & Roberts, T. B. (Eds.). (2007). Psychedelic medicine: New evidence for hallucinogenic substances as treatments, Volume 1 & 2. Westport, CT: Praeger.

292. Wolfe, B. E., & Mott, J. H. (2017). The Integration of Psychological Principles in Policy Development. Contributions to Psychology, 1-15.

293. Wolfe, J. D., & Thornhill, L. P. (2021). The Renaissance of Psychedelic Psychiatry. The Canadian Journal of Psychiatry, 66(2).

294. Wollinsky, H., Asher, Y., Bekier, E., & Berger, U. (2018). Rapid and longer-term antidepressant effects of repeated ketamine infusions in treatment-resistant major depression. Biological Psychiatry, 84(4), 265-276.

295. Yaden, D. B., Griffiths, R. R., & Zauner, N. (2021). The subjective effects of psychedelics are necessary for their enduring therapeutic effects. ACS Pharmacology & Translational Science, 4(2), 568-572.

296. Yazar-Klosinski, B. B., & Mithoefer, M. C. (2017). Potential psychiatric uses for MDMA. Clinical Pharmacology & Therapeutics, 101(2), 194-196.

297. Yehuda, R., & LeDoux, J. (2007). Response variation following trauma: A translational neuroscience approach to understanding PTSD. Neuron, 56(1), 19-32.

298. Zarate, C. A., Singh, J. B., Carlson, P. J., Brutsche, N. E., Ameli, R., Luckenbaugh, D. A., ... & Manji, H. K. (2006). A randomized trial of an N-methyl-D-aspartate antagonist in treatment-resistant major depression. Archives of General Psychiatry, 63(8), 856-864.

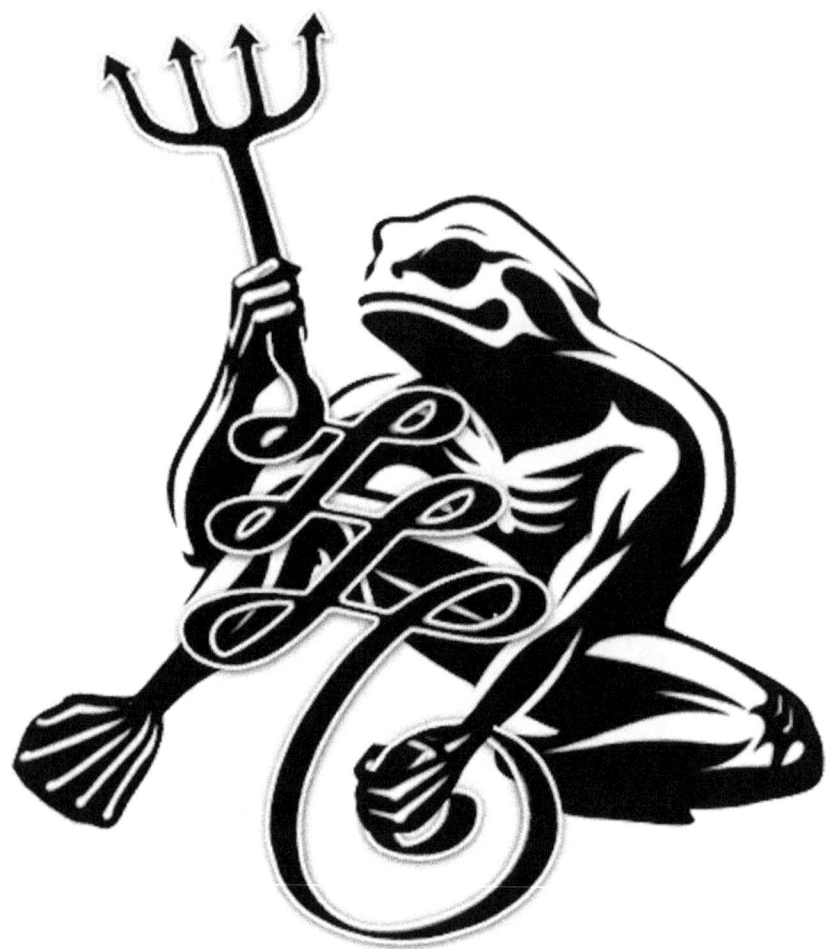

www.ingramcontent.com/pod-product-compliance
Lightning Source LLC
Chambersburg PA
CBHW072046020426
42334CB00017B/1411